An Atlas of ATOPIC ECZEMA

THE ENCYCLOPEDIA OF VISUAL MEDICINE SERIES

An Atlas of ATOPIC ECZEMA

Lionel Fry, BSC, MD, FRCP
Professor Emeritus of Dermatology
Imperial College
London, UK
Foreword by

Charles N.Ellis, MD
Professor and Associate Chair
Department of Dermatology
University of Michigan, USA

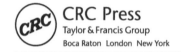

CRC Press
Taylor & Francis Group
Boca Raton London New York

CRC Press is an imprint of the
Taylor & Francis Group, an **informa** business

Published in the USA by
The Parthenon Publishing Group Inc.
345 Park Avenue South, 10th Floor
New York
NY 10010
USA

Published in the UK and Europe by
The Parthenon Publishing Group
23–25 Blades Court
Deodar Road
London SW15 2NU
UK

Library of Congress Cataloging-in-Publication Data
Fry, Lionel.
An atlas of atopic eczema/Lionel Fry.
p. ; cm. —(The encyclopedia of visual medicine series)
Includes bibliographical references and index.
ISBN 1-84214-236-4 (hard cover : alk paper)
1. Atopic dermatitis-Atlases. I.Title: Atopic eczema. II. Title. III. Series
[DNLM: 1. Dermatitis, Atopic-Atlases. WR 17 F946ab 2003]
RC593.A8F79 2003
616.5'1–dc22

British Library Cataloguing in Publication Data
Fry, Lionel, 1933–
An atlas of atopic eczema.—[The encyclopedia of visual
medicine series)
1. Atopic dermatitis
I. Title
616.5'21

ISBN 0-203-49050-9 Master e-book ISBN

ISBN 0-203-59659-5 (Adobe eReader Format)
ISBN 1-84214-236-4 (Print Edition)

First published in 2004

This edition published in the Taylor & Francis e-Library, 2005.

"To purchase your own copy of this or any of Taylor & Francis or Routledge's collection of
thousands of eBooks please go to www.eBookstore.tandf.co.uk."

Composition by The Parthenon Publishing Group

Contents

Foreword — vii

Preface — viii

1 Definitions — 1
Dermatitis versus eczema — 1
Atopic — 1
Infantile eczema — 2

2 Epidemiology — 3
Place of domicile — 3
Incidence of atopic eczema related to age — 3
Increasing incidence of atopic eczema — 3

3 Natural history — 4

4 Genetics — 6
Family studies — 6
Twin studies — 6
Human lymphocyte antigen system — 6
Genome screens — 6
Maternal effect — 7
Summary — 7

5 Pathogenesis — 8
Histology — 8
Findings in the blood — 8
Immunopathogenesis — 10
Inflammatory cells — 11
Immunoglobulin E — 12
Summary — 12

6 Etiology — 13
Genetics: possible candidate genes — 13
Abnormal skin barrier — 14
Allergens — 15
Aeroallergens — 15
Autoantigens — 16

Bacteria 16

Fungi 18

Environmental pollution 18

Hygiene hypothesis 18

Pharmacological and vascular abnormalities 20

Emotional factors 20

Neuropeptides 21

Summary 21

7   Clinical features 22

Age of onset 22

Sex 22

Clinical features of eczema *per* se 22

Age-related features 22

Non-age-related features 24

Atopic eczema at specific sites 26

Other eczematous skin disorders in atopic individuals 29

Non-eczematous cutaneous features of atopy 30

Other disorders associated with atopic eczema 31

Infections 33

8   Differential diagnosis 81

Other eczematous conditions 81

Syndromes with eczematous eruptions 82

Non-eczema disorders 83

9   Management 91

Emollients 91

Bathing 91

Clothing 91

Climate 91

Diet 92

Breast-feeding 92

Delayed introduction of solid foods 92

Avoidance of food antigens in pregnancy 92

Probiotics 92

Aeroallergens 93

Animals 93

Psychotherapeutic measures 93

Investigations 93

Topical drugs 93

Antistaphylococcal treatment 98

Antiviral treatment 98

Antifungal treatment 98

Ultraviolet light 98

Systemic treatment 99

Biological agents 100

The future 100

References 101

Index 103

Foreword

A picture shows me at a glance what it takes dozens of pages of a book to expound.

Ivan Sergeyevich Turgenev, 1862

In this slim but focused book, Professor Lionel Fry has captured all we need to know about eczema. Akin to the quote above, proverbially one picture is worth more than 10 000 words. This Atlas is replete with diagrams, helpful reminders in illustrative form, and plenty of pictures of the many expressions of eczema. The teachings of the renowned Professor Fry are delightfully presented in both word and illustration.

This book is timely because of the new information that has developed recently, particularly with regard to the pathogenesis of eczema (Chapters 5 and 6) and the treatments that are newly available or are coming shortly (Chapter 9). Just sit with this book for an hour or two, and one will feel on top of the challenge of the eczemas. I invite you to take advantage of Professor Fry's great knowledge in this area and his clarity of writing. The eczemas, which were so mysterious before, have the veil of confusion lifted in this Atlas.

The excellent pictures and the accompanying text will be of great value to all who diagnose and treat skin diseases, including dermatologists, general practitioners, pediatricians, internists, gynecologists, and, for that matter, any physician or nurse with family or friends who seek advice about skin disorders. The eczemas, which are so common, are increasing in incidence, and therefore all of us must be cognizant of their various presentations and treatment.

Charles N.Ellis, MD
Professor and Associate Chair
Department of Dermatology
University of Michigan
Ann Arbor, 2004

Preface

Atopic eczema is still one of the major problems in the field of dermatology. The rising incidence has been attributed to a number of factors including increasing urbanization, pollution and the 'hygiene hypothesis'. The latter attributes the increase in atopy as being due to a decline of infections in early life, related to the use of antibiotics and immunizations and to smaller families.

Over the last few years, advances have been made in the genetics of atopy in general; newer treatments have been introduced for topical use and new concepts suggested in the etiology. Thus, a new text on atopic eczema seems timely.

Atopic eczema presents to general practitioners, pediatricians, dermatologists and allergists and, therefore, I hope that this book will be of value to physicians in these fields, particularly those in training. The ample illustrations are intended to help in the diagnosis and management of this common complaint.

I am grateful to Mr Bruce Mathalone for the use of illustrations on eye conditions associated with atopy and to Dr Nick Francis for the histology illustrations. I am also pleased to acknowledge the contributions of Zachary Fry and the endeavours of my secretary, Mrs Helen Morris Crawshaw.

Lionel Fry

1
Definitions

DERMATITIS VERSUS ECZEMA

The words 'dermatitis' and 'eczema' are used synonymously in the dermatological literature. Dermatitis derives from the Greek word *derma,* meaning skin. However, the word 'dermis' is now applied to the structure of the skin below the basement membrane, whilst that above is called the epidermis. Thus, it could be argued that dermatitis, strictly speaking, refers to the dermis and not to the whole skin. Eczema is derived from the Greek word *ekzein,* meaning 'to boil over', and is a purely descriptive term. Which term is more accurate is debatable. In this book, the term eczema is preferred, but the choice is arbitrary.

ATOPIC

The word 'atopic' is derived from the Greek word *topos,* meaning place, and was applied in the sense 'out of place'. The term was coined to denote an abnormal hypersensitive response to an environmental allergen and the word 'atopen' is now synonymous with allergen. Two allergists, Coco and Cooke, first used the term 'atopic' in 1923[1], and the term 'atopic dermatitis' originated in 1933. However, the condition that is now described by this term is considerably older and can be recognized in early Chinese and Roman writings.

At present, there is no universal agreement about the definition of atopic eczema. Some believe that immunoglobulin E (IgE)-specific antibodies to environmental antigens are part of the disease and the term atopic eczema should not be used if IgE allergen-specific antibodies are not present[2]. If the clinical features suggest atopic eczema but no IgE antibodies are present, the term 'atopiform' eczema has been proposed[2]. Others believe that atopic eczema defines a clinical state with characteristic features. The clinical criteria postulated by Hanifin and Rajka[3] are still the most appropriate. They give four major features, of which at least three must be present. These are:

(1) Pruritus;
(2) Lichenification;
(3) Chronic relapsing course;
(4) Personal and/or family history of asthma, allergic rhinitis/conjunctivitis and a family history of atopic eczema.

In addition, three minor features should be present. These include dryness of the skin, ichthyosis vulgaris, keratosis pilaris, immediate skin test (type 1) reactivity, elevated IgE level, tendency to cutaneous infection with *Staphylococcus aureus* and herpes simplex, increased incidence of hand and foot and nipple eczema, cheilitis, recurrent conjunctivitis, Dennie-Morgan infraorbital fold, anterior subcapsular cataracts, orbital darkening, facial pallor/erythema, pityriasis alba, anterior neck folds, itch when sweating, intolerance to wool, perifollicular accentuation, food intolerance, course often affected by emotional/environmental factors, and white dermographism.

More simple criteria were proposed by Williams and colleagues[4]. These are: a history of an itchy skin rash in the last 12 months plus three or more of the following:

(1) History of flexural involvement;
(2) History of asthma and/or hay fever;
(3) History of generalized dry skin;
(4) Onset of rash before the age of 2 years (not applicable if the patient is under 4 years);
(5) Visible flexural involvement.

These criteria are not as precise as those of Hanifin and Rajka and may not be applicable to young children and infants.

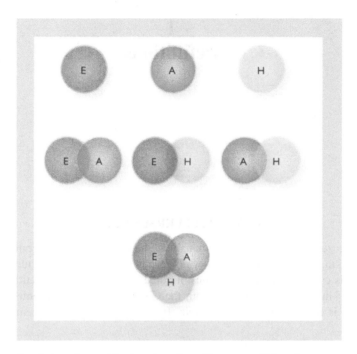

Figure 1 Atopic disease may occur singularly or in combination. A, asthma; E, eczema; H, hay fever

It should be remembered that 100% uniformity does not exist in clinical medicine and there are always exceptions to the clinical criteria as proposed both by Hanifin and Rajka, and by Williams and colleagues.

A causative role for IgE antibodies in atopic eczema is still disputed and other pathogenetic mechanisms have been implicated. Until these have been fully elucidated, it would be prudent to maintain the clinical criteria for diagnosing atopic eczema.

IgE antibodies are found in 70–80% of patients with atopic eczema. The terms 'intrinsic' and 'extrinsic' have been used to imply that evidence exists for an external allergen based on IgE antibodies. The term 'extrinsic atopic eczema' is used when antibodies are present and 'intrinsic' when the antibodies are absent. How useful this subdivision is at the clinical level is debatable at present but, with greater understanding of the pathogenesis of atopic eczema in the future, this subdivision may then be relevant.

Atopic eczema is strongly associated with asthma, rhinitis and conjunctivitis, due to external allergens. However, as with eczema, the demonstration that the disease is due to an external allergen is not always proven. Asthma is also divided into intrinsic and extrinsic subdivisions. Collectively, eczema, asthma and hay fever are sometimes referred to as the atopic syndrome. However, it is important to stress that the three manifestations of the atopic syndrome may occur singularly and not necessarily all together (Figure 1).

INFANTILE ECZEMA

Atopic eczema is sometimes still referred to as infantile or flexural eczema because of its early age of onset and the characteristic sites of the disease. However, the term 'atopic eczema' is to be preferred because other types of eczema may occur in infancy and may affect flexures. In addition, there are prognostic and genetic implications associated with atopic eczema that are different from the other patterns of eczema seen in childhood.

2
Epidemiology

PLACE OF DOMICILE

Epidemiological studies on atopic eczema have been carried out, particularly in European countries. However, the accuracy of these studies is dependent on the definitions of atopic eczema that were used, and the fact that many are based on questionnaires rather than on an interview and examination by a dermatologist. There are also variations in the questions posed and the age of the groups studied. Thus, some studies have only taken the incidence of eczema at a particular point in time and others have included past history.

Using point prevalence (i.e. presence of eczema at that particular point), the incidence of the disease in European countries ranges from 5.3 to 26%, with a mean of 13% in the groups aged 3–12 years[5]. In one of the largest studies conducted world-wide, questionnaires were completed on 458 623 individuals, aged 13–14 years. The incidence of atopic eczema ranged from more than 15% in some northern European countries to less than 5% in China, central Asia and eastern European countries[6]. There was a suggestion that the line of latitude had an effect in that the closer to the equator the country was, the lower the incidence of the disease. However, it is interesting to note that, when individuals migrate from areas of low incidence to those of a higher incidence, the incidence of atopic eczema rises in the immigrant population and is often higher than in the local population. Thus, environmental factors are of considerable importance in determining the incidence of atopic eczema. In addition, an increased incidence of the disease appears to be associated with a move from a rural/agricultural society to an industrial one. It has been shown, in a study in Ibadan in Nigeria, that the incidence of atopic eczema increased with the progressive industrialization of the area and an associated change in lifestyle. Thus, change in lifestyle may be more important than the change in the latitude of the country of residence.

INCIDENCE OF ATOPIC ECZEMA RELATED TO AGE

It is generally agreed that the incidence of atopic eczema decreases as children become older and the incidence is considerably less in adult life. As already mentioned, the incidence of atopic eczema in northern European countries is relatively high in children, particularly in urban areas. Several studies give an incidence of 10–15% and most of these studies are for the age group 3–11 years[7]. The studies do not distinguish between the incidences at age 3 and age 11. A few studies have examined the incidences in the 0–4–year age group, where they ranged from approximately 10 to 15%. Studies in teenagers have shown considerably lower incidences in the same countries and these range from approximately 2 to 3%. The frequency in adults is even lower; over the age of 25, the incidence has been reported to be less than 0.2%[8]. Thus, to inform parents that children usually grow out of their eczema is correct.

INCREASING INCIDENCE OF ATOPIC ECZEMA

It has been thought that the incidence of atopic eczema has increased over the last 50 years. However, the figures supporting this observation may not be reliable because of the criteria and techniques used to arrive at these results. The criteria for diagnosing atopic eczema and the concept of the disease have changed over time. Many of the figures are based on parents' recall of the rash in their children and no objective examinations were carried out in most of the studies. If these limitations are accepted, then the figures do show an increasing incidence of atopic eczema in children. In children up to 7 years, the incidence for those born before 1960 ranged from 1.4 to 3.1%, with a mean of 2.2%. For those born between 1960 and 1970, the frequency ranged from 3.8 to 8.8%, with a mean of 6.7%, and, for those born after 1970, the range was 8.9–20.4%, with a mean of 12.0%[9]. This increased incidence of atopic eczema is supported by twin studies from Denmark. The cumulative incidence rate for twins born between 1960 and 1964 was 3% and for those born between 1975 and 1979 it rose to 12%[10].

This increase in the incidence of atopic eczema is similar to the reported increase in asthma seen over the last 40 years.

3
Natural history

Although there have been several studies on the natural history of atopic eczema, there are a number of variable factors in these studies that may influence their reliability. First, the definition of the disease was not consistent. Second, the length of time of follow-up was variable. Third, some of the studies were hospital-based while others were community-based. It is likely that community-based studies will show milder disease than a hospital-based population and the severity of the disease may influence the natural history.

It is generally agreed that atopic eczema usually commences in childhood. In nearly 50% of patients, the age of onset is before 6 months, with 60% before 1 year and 70% before 5 years[11]. It is also accepted that atopic eczema will go into remission in early life. In a general practice setting over a 40-year study period, it was found that 50% of cases had cleared by the age of 5 years and 90% by the age of 10 (J. Fry, personal communication). In a British cohort study, 65% had cleared by age 11 and 74% by age 16[12]. In a hospital-based study over a 5–20-year period, the clearance rates ranged from 84 to 92%[13]. Thus, there is general agreement that atopic eczema is primarily a disease of childhood, with the majority clearing before or during adolescence. However, in a smaller proportion, atopic eczema may present for the first time in adult life, and in some individuals, whose eczema began in infancy, the disease will persist into adult life. The factors that determine these variations are yet to be elucidated but; similar to the basic causes of the disease, they are likely to be partly constitutional and partly environmental. It is also well known that, in patients whose atopic eczema has cleared, there is always a risk that it may recur because of inherent factors. Occupations and hobbies in later life, involving exposure to chemicals that may damage the stratum corneum, may induce eczematous reactions, either for the first time or as a recurrence in those with a past history of atopic eczema.

Various factors have been implicated in a poor prognosis. These include severe disease at onset; extensor or inverse pattern of eczema on the knees and elbows in children; family history of atopic eczema, particularly if both parents are affected; concomitant asthma; and subjects who were not breast-fed. However, these are also studies disputing these factors as poor prognostic indicators.

The risk of developing asthma and hay fever in children with atopic eczema has been reported in a number of studies[14]. The main criticisms of these studies are that the period of study was too short or that the subjects were chosen from a hospital-based population, thus implying a disease more severe than in the true spectrum of atopic eczema severity. The periods of

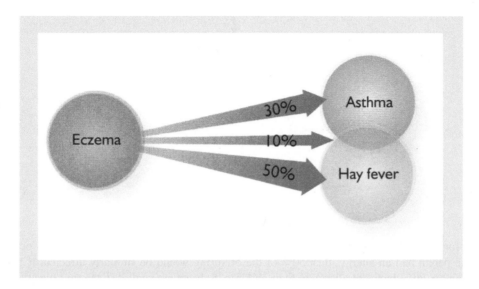

Figure 2 Approximate percentages of atopic eczema individuals who subsequently develop asthma and/or hay fever

study have mostly been 5–15 years and the incidence of asthma has ranged from 10 to 53% and that for hay fever from 28 to 78%. In one large study[15], in which patients were traced after 22–44 years, the incidence of asthma was 37% for patients who were inpatients and 22% in those who were outpatients; for hay fever, the figures were 66% for inpatients and 33% for outpatients. The two main findings of these studies are that the risk of developing hay fever is greater than that of developing asthma (Figure 2) and that the more severe the eczema, the greater the likelihood of developing asthma and hay fever.

4
Genetics

FAMILY STUDIES

It has been known for nearly 100 years that 'allergy' runs in families. Original studies in 1916 by Cooke and Van der Veer reported that, if one parent had an allergy, then 50% of the offspring would be similarly affected; if both parents had an a allergy, then there was a 75% chance of allergy in their children. Subsequent studies in the mid-twentieth century concluded that genetic factors were more important than environmental ones in atopic disorders. All types of Mendelian inheritance were proposed, but, by the 1960s, it was generally agreed that atopic disorders were polygenic (several genes involved) and that the diseases were multifactorial (in other words, environmental as well as genetic factors were implicated).

If one considers asthma, hay fever (allergic rhinitis) and eczema as constituting the 'atopic diathesis', then; in patients with atopic eczema, those with a positive family history of atopy have been reported as ranging from 43 to 83%, with a mean of approximately 60–65%. It is well known that, although the individual patient may present with eczema, the affected relatives may have asthma, allergic rhinitis or eczema. However, there is usually a higher incidence of the presenting disease in the family of the proband, i.e. if the presenting disease is asthma, then there is a higher incidence, in the family, of asthma compared to eczema and hay fever. The same is true for eczema and hay fever. This has led to the concept of 'end-organ sensitivity' and the genetic determinants for variants of atopic diathesis do appear to run in families.

TWIN STUDIES

To determine the role of genetic factors in multifactorial disorders, twin studies have proved helpful in determining the importance of genetic influence. The most recent figures for twins with atopic eczema show a concordance rate of 75% for monozygotic and 20% for dizygotic twins[16]. These figures imply a strong genetic component for atopic eczema and, interestingly, are very similar to those for psoriasis, another common inflammatory dermatosis.

HUMAN LYMPHOCYTE ANTIGEN SYSTEM

Immunological factors would appear to play an important role in atopic eczema and therefore, the human lymphocyte antigen (HLA) system, which is associated with immune responses, would be expected to show certain HLA antigens associated with atopic eczema. However, despite a number of studies, no specific HLA antigen or haplotype has been found to be associated with atopic eczema. This lack of association is supported by the genome scans that have been performed in atopic eczema in which no loci have been reported on chromosome 6p, which is where the HLA region is found. Interestingly, in asthma, linkage to chromosome 6p has been reported and also a significant increase in the HLA haplotype B7, SC31, DR2 has been found. This implies that the immune mechanisms in asthma and atopic eczema may not have common pathways.

GENOME SCREENS

To date, two genome screens have been performed in atopic eczema in childhood and one in adults[17]. In the first, performed in children in a German and Scandinavian population, linkage was found to chromosome 3q21. In the second, in British families, linkage was found to 1q21, 17q25, and 20p. The latter study included some individuals with asthma as well as atopic eczema. Interestingly, in the German and Scandinavian study, linkage to the total serum IgE level was also found with the 3q21 locus but the British study found linkage for the IgE level to chromosomes 5q31 and 16qtel.

In the one adult study, on Swedish individuals, linkage was reported for chromosome 3p24–22. If the IgE level was included as a trait, then linkage to 18q21 was found. When the severity scores of the eczema were included, the suggested linkage to chromosomes 3q14, 13q14, 15q14–15, and 17q21 was found. Thus, the only common linkage for adults and children was 17q21 and possibly on chromosome 3q. The implication of these findings is that different pathogenic mechanisms may be operative in childhood and in adult atopic eczema.

When these results on genome screens are compared to those for asthma, differences are found. The agreed loci for asthma are 5q35, 6p, 11q13, 12q, 13q13, 14q and 16q. Interestingly, there are very few common loci for the two disorders; the only possible areas so far are 13q and 16q, but the regions reported are not the same. The implication of these findings is that different pathogenic mechanisms are operative in the two diseases, as suggested by the HLA findings.

Recently, it has been pointed out that similar loci have been reported (1q21, 17q15 and 20p) for psoriasis and atopic eczema, which are both inflammatory skin diseases[18]. Thus, these associations may be related to the control of inflammation in the skin and not to the basic causes of the diseases.

IgE has been implicated in the pathogenesis of atopic diseases because there are increased levels in the serum in approximately 75% of patients. Atopic asthma has been linked to a locus on chromosome 11q12–13, where a gene controlling the subunit of the high-affinity receptor for IgE (FceRI) is localized. Linkage to 11q12–13 has not been reported in genome screens in atopic eczema, but there is a report of an association of atopic eczema and the   unit of FceR1 in that polymorphisms within this unit are strongly associated with atopic eczema[19]. This paradox has not been resolved as yet.

MATERNAL EFFECT

It has been noted in a number of studies that mothers are more likely to transmit atopic disorders, including eczema, than fathers[20]. There are a number of possible reasons for this observation. First, there is a close association between the maternal and fetal immune systems, and interactions between the two might influence the development of the fetal immune system, and its response to external stimuli. The second possibility is that of genome imprinting in which the allele from one parent is differentially expressed. However, it has been found that the maternal linkage to atopic disease is not confined to a single genetic mechanism at one single gene locus[21].

SUMMARY

Thus, there is strong evidence for a genetic component in the etiology of atopic eczema. However, considering that immune mechanisms are involved in the pathogenesis, it should be noted that, as yet, there is no association with a particular HLA haplotype. In addition, despite the close association between asthma and atopic eczema, there is to date no common genotype for the two disorders.

5
Pathogenesis

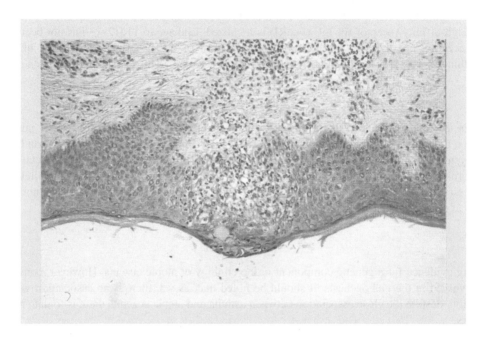

Figure 3 Acute eczema with spongiosis in the epidermis and a dermal infiltrate of inflammatory cells, mainly lymphocytes and macrophages

HISTOLOGY

The histological features of atopic eczema vary, depending on whether the disease is acute, subacute or chronic

In the *acute* phase, spongiosis progressing to blister formation is the characteristic feature. Spongiosis is defined as an increase in the amount of tissue fluid between the keratinocytes in the epidermis, which is visible as a widening of the intercellular space (Figure 3). Some intracellular edema also occurs. Lymphocytes migrate through the epidermis (exocytosis) and there is a perivascular infiltrate of lymphocytes and macrophages into the dermis but with no increase in number of mast cells or basophils. However, the mast cells are in various stages of degranulation, indicating activation. Occasionally, eosinophils are present.

In the *subacute* phase, the epidermis begins to thicken and the spongiosis lessens.

In the *chronic* phase, the epidermis is thick (Figures 4 and 5) and similar in appearance to the epidermis in psoriasis, but the 'folding' of the interphase between the dermis and epidermis,   present in psoriasis, is not seen in atopic eczema. The thickening is caused by hyperplasia of the keratinocytes. The dermis is infiltrated by mast cells, lymphocytes and eosinophils (Figure 4). As in psoriasis, the blood vessels in the dermis become more prominent. Langerhans and dendritic cells are increased in number in both the epidermis and dermis. The chronic phase (Figure 5) is often associated with persistent scratching and this has been linked to changes in the cutaneous nerves, which show demyelination, vacuolation and fibrosis.

FINDINGS IN THE BLOOD

So-called 'reagenic' antibodies in the blood of patients with atopic disease were first demonstrated by Prausnitz and Kustner in 1921[22]. These have now been shown to be IgE antibodies to foreign protein, which may be antigenic in atopics. Approximately 75–80% of patients with atopic eczema have raised IgE levels and blood eosinophilia also occurs. Peripheral blood

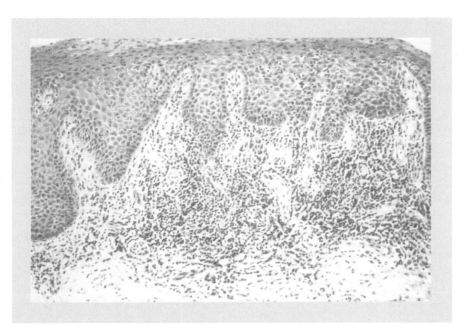

Figure 4 Chronic phase of eczema with thickening of the epidermis and an intense infiltrate in the dermis of mast cells, lymphocytes, eosinophils and dendritic cells

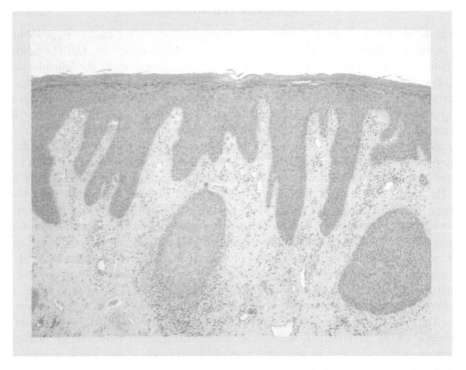

Figure 5 Lichen simplex: chronic atopic eczema associated with continual scratching. There is more accentuation of the rete pegs of the epidermis

mononuclear cells have a decreased ability to produce interferon-gamma (IFN-), the levels of which are inversely correlated with those of IgE. However, there is an increase in allergen-specific lymphocytes producing the cytokines inter-leukin IL-4, IL-5, and IL-13. These are the cytokines that are capable of inducing IgE production (Figure 6). These cytokines also induce expression of vascular adhesion molecules, for example, VCAM-1, which are involved in eosinophilic infiltrations of the skin. These findings reflect the inverse relationship between T-helper cells types 1 and 2 (Th1 and Th2) and their respective cytokines. Th1 cells produce IFN- , which down-regulates the production of IL-4 and IL-5 by Th2 cells. Conversely, the IL-4 and Il-5 cytokines down-regulate production of IFN- by Th1 cells (Figure 6). In atopic eczema, there is a shift in favor of Th2 cells and their cytokines. In addition, IL-5 activates the production of eosino-phils, a characteristic feature of atopy.

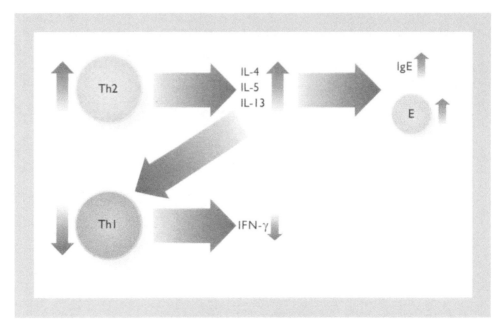

Figure 6 In atopic eczema, there is an increase in blood of the Th2 cells producing IL-4, IL-5, IL-13 and an associated increase in IgE. Production of IFN- by Th1 cells is decreased. E, eosinophil

IMMUNOPATHOGENESIS

The eczematous response in the skin in atopic eczema is a T-lymphocyte-mediated disorder (type IV hypersensitivity) and is antigen-dependent. In theory, the antigen could be inhaled, ingested or enter through the skin. The inhaled or ingested antigen may enter the circulation and be carried to the lymph nodes, where it is picked up by the follicular dendritic cells, antigen-presenting cells and B-cells. The follicular dendritic cells present the antigen to T-cells, which can then induce the B-cells to produce IgE. This process will continue for the period in which allergen-specific T- and B-cells remain in the lymph nodes.

The method by which the ingested or inhaled allergen enters the skin is subject to debate. However, once the allergen is in the skin, it can be picked up by IgE receptors on Langerhans cells, which are antigen-presenting cells.

One of the characteristic features of atopic eczema is the IgE receptor on the Langerhans cells in the skin. The expression of this receptor may possibly be under genetic control. The antigen that arrives in the skin and binds to the IgE receptor will then be processed and presented to the T-lymphocytes in the skin. In the acute stage of atopic eczema, cytokine production is of the Th2 profile. The Th2 cytokines are IL-4, IL-5 and IL-13 (Figure 7). However, in the chronic phase of atopic eczema, there is a switch from a Th2 to a Th1 cytokine profile by the lymphocytes (Figure 7). Thus, the hypothesis that atopic eczema is a Th2 response to antigen, as opposed to a Th1 response, is not strictly correct because both responses can happen. In the so-called atopic patch test, when eczema is induced by application of house-dust allergen, a biphasic response occurs. In the first instance, there is a Th2 response with mainly IL-4 production, but, after 24 h, there is a Th1 response with IFN-production. Thus, atopic individuals are able to mount both Th1 and Th2 immune responses and the concept that the responses are mutually exclusive is only correct for a given point in time. Thoughts on the factors that govern the switch from a Th2 to a Th1 response in atopic eczema are speculative. It has been suggested that both cytokines IL-12 and IL-18 can induce a shift from a Th2 to a Th1 response[23]. IL-12 is produced by constitutive cells of the skin, keratinocytes, dendritic cells and dermal macrophages and by the infiltrating cells, i.e. eosinophils (Figure 7). However, the mechanism that controls the inhi-bition/production of these cytokines in the acute and chronic phases of the atopic eczema state requires further elucidation. It does appear that the initial response to antigen in atopy is Th2-mediated but, subsequently, in the more chronic phase, it is Th1-mediated. The argument that what is required to cure atopic eczema is to shift the immune response from a Th2 to a Th1 response is thus only partly correct, since, in the chronic phase, it is a Th1 response. However, the initiation is likely to be via a Th2 mechanism, so a permanent switch to a Th1 response may be helpful in clearing the eczema more permanently.

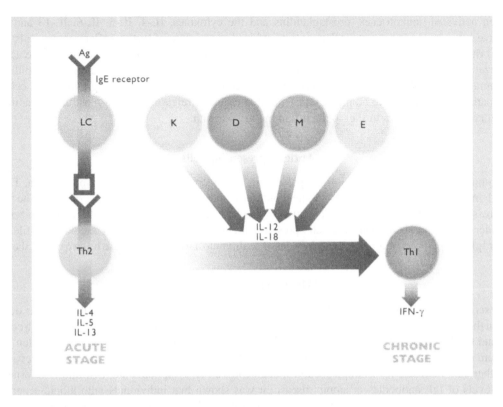

Figure 7 Cytokine production in the skin in atopic eczema. Ag, antigen; LC, Langerhans cells; K, keratinocyte; D, dendritic cells; M, dermal macrophages; E, eosinophil

INFLAMMATORY CELLS

T-lymphocytes

In atopic eczema, there is an influx of predominantly CD4+ in the dermis and epidermis. The number of T-cells in the skin correlates with the level of IL-16, which is a chemoattractant for CD4 T-cells. IL-16 is produced by eosinophils, mast cells and T-cells and, thus, these activated T-cells can maintain the inflammatory process.

Some of the T-cells in the skin express CD45RO, which is a marker of activated/memory T-cells, meaning that they are primed to react to specific antigens. CD8+ T-cells have received little attention in atopic eczema but they can be found in the infiltrate. It was originally considered that CD8 T-cells had a suppressor role, but they have been shown, in addition, to be effector cells.

Eosinophils

Increased numbers of eosinophils in the blood and affected tissues are a feature of atopic diseases. Chemotaxis of eosinophils into the skin is related to the C-C chemokines, eotaxin and monocyte chemotactic 4, which are increased in atopic eczema. Activation of the eosinophils is induced by cytokines granulocyte-macrophage colony stimulating factors (GM-CSF), IL-5 and eotaxin. Once activated, the eosinophils may promote inflammation and tissue damage by the release of various chemicals, including eosinophilic cation protein, major basic protein, eosinophilic derived neurotoxin, and reactive oxygen species.

Mast cells

Mast cells are present in the skin of patients with atopic eczema. They have IgE receptors on their cell surface but their exact role in atopic eczema is not certain.

Mast cells are most commonly activated by their IgE receptors and, once activated, the cells degranulate. They release a variety of products connected with inflammation. The preferred mast cell products, which can be released on activation, include heparin, histamine, serotonin, chymase, tryptase and tumor necrosis factor-alpha (TNF-). The mast cells also synthesize, when activated, leukotrienes, prostaglandins and the cytokines, IL-4, IL-5, IL-6, IL-13 and GM-CSF. These biologically active substances can promote inflammation and lead to an influx of further inflammatory cells into the skin.

In asthma and rhinitis, mast cell degranulation occurs at an early stage and is probably involved in the acute inflammatory responses. In eczema, however, the mast cells are deep in the skin (dermis) in contrast to being in the epithelium of the nose and lung in asthma and rhinitis where they are thus easily accessible to allergens. It is thought that mast cell degranulation is not part of the pathological process in atopic eczema, but that cytokine release from the mast cells, leading to an influx of other inflammatory cells, contributes further to the inflammatory reaction.

Antigen-presenting cells

As with other immune cells, the number of antigen-presenting cells (APC) is increased in atopic eczema. These cells include Langerhans and inflammatory dendritic cells in the epidermis and dendritic cells in the dermis. The Langerhans cells exclusively express IgE receptors, a characteristic feature of atopic disease, and present antigens to T-cells with a Th2 cytokine profile. The epidermal inflammatory dendritic cells present antigen to T-cells with a Th1 cytokine profile. The Langerhans cells positive for IgE receptors can migrate to lymph nodes and stimulate naïve T-cells, there by expanding the pool of Th2 cells.

IMMUNOGLOBULIN E

IgE was first described in 1967 and the radioallergosorbent test (RAST) for specific IgE antibodies was developed in 1971. IgE is elevated in the serum in 75–80% of patients with atopic eczema, and it has been claimed that there is a correlation between the IgE levels and the severity of the eczema. However, it has to be remembered that IgE levels are often raised in subjects not suffering from eczema and there are patients with atopic eczema who have normal levels of IgE. Elevated IgE levels are also found in other skin diseases, for example, scabies, cutaneous T-cell lymphoma and helminthic infestations. In a recent study[24] on the levels of IgE antibodies in atopic disease, it was shown that individuals with atopic eczema have 20 times higher levels of antibodies to house dust mites than those with atopic asthma, even though the house dust mite is considered to be an aeroallergen for asthma. Thus, the significance of this high level of IgE in eczema needs to be explained.

IgE is produced by B-cells and is thought to be under the control of IL-4. Atopic eczema is characterized by Th2 cells which produce IL-4. This, in turn, may stimulate IgE production. It is possible, therefore, that the elevated IgE level is secondary to this process and may not have an initiating role in this eczematous process. Thus, a role for IgE and its antibodies has yet to be defined.

SUMMARY

Atopic eczema is an inflammatory skin condition that is antigen-driven and T-cell-mediated. The two typical features are the presence of IgE receptors on Langerhans cells and a Th2 cytokine profile in the acute stages. However, in the chronic phase, there is a Th1 cytokine profile with IFN- production that down-regulates IgE production and Th2 lymphocytes.

It should be remembered that not all patients with atopic eczema have raised serum IgE levels. Whether the pathogenetic mechanisms in these individuals are the same as those in patients with raised serum IgE levels is yet to be elucidated.

6
Etiology

GENETICS: POSSIBLE CANDIDATE GENES

As discussed in Chapter 4, the role of genetic factors is important in atopic eczema and a number of chromosome loci have been implicated.

Chromosome 3q21

This region encodes for the co-stimulating molecules CD80 and CD86; a mutation in these genes could lead to an alteration in T-cell activation.

Chromosome 5q31

The locus 5q31 contains the gene SPINK5, which has recently been identified as the gene for Netherton's syndrome. Netherton's syndrome is an autosomal recessive disorder, which includes the atopic manifestations of eczema, hay fever, eosinophilia and high serum IgE levels. SPINK5 was so named as it encodes for an enzyme inhibitor, 'serine proteinase inhibitor, Kazal type 5'. The serine proteinase inhibitor has been termed LEKTI, as it is found in the lymphoid tissue of the thymus and epithelial tissue, including skin. (The KT is kazal type and I is inhibitor.)

Recently, six coding polymorphisms in SPINK5 have been identified; a GLu 420   Lys variant shows significant association with atopy and atopic eczema[25]. This abnormality in the proteinase inhibitor may influence allergic disease. Proteinase activated receptors are found in keratinocytes and can serve as targets for mast cell proteinases. Proteinases are involved in the maturation of T- and B-cells and the expression of LEKTI in the thymus may suggest a role for these processes in allergic diseases. In addition, many allergens are serine proteinases and this proteinase activity may encourage their allergenicity in the presence of defective inhibition.

SPINK5 also lies in the region where the cluster of cytokine genes, particularly Th2 cytokines, IL-4, IL-5, and IL-13, is found. These Th2 cytokines are implicated in atopic eczema.

Chromosome 11q13

This region was originally linked to atopic asthma and eczema. It contains a gene that is associated with polymorphism of the -chain of the high-affinity receptor for IgE (FceRI). This receptor acts as an allergic trigger on mast cells and basophils, leading to intracellular degranulation of these cells and the associated release of inflammatory mediators, which have a role in asthma and hay fever. In addition, IgE receptors are present on antigen-presenting cells and have been implicated in the pathogenesis of atopic eczema. However, it has recently been reported that the FceRI on antigen-presenting cells lacks the classical -chain, although the receptor has full function[26]. Thus; although the gene controlling the -subunit of FceRI may be important in atopic asthma and rhinitis, it may not have a role in eczema.

Chromosome 13q14

Recently, it has been shown that serum IgE levels are related to alleles in the gene *PHF11* in asthma. It is thought that this gene regulates IgE production by B-cells in atopic disease[27].

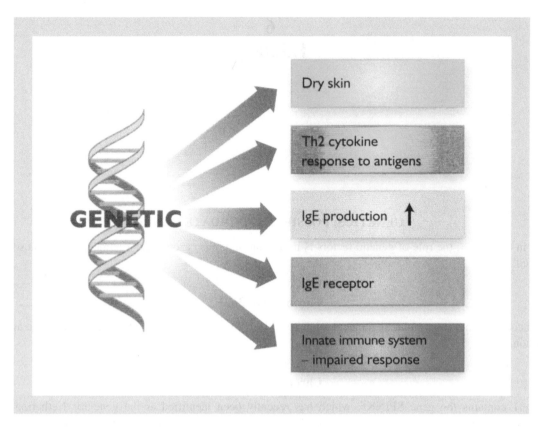

Figure 8 Possible genetic abnormalities in atopic eczema

Chromosome 16q12

This locus has been linked to polymorphism in the -subunit of the IL-4 receptor. IL-4 is considered to have a central role in atopic eczema.

Chromosome 17q11

Atopic eczema is associated with up-regulation of C-C chemokine expression. RANTES (regulated-on-activation normal T-cell, expressed and secreted) is a member of the C-C chemokine family and is considered to play a central role in allergic inflammation. A single polymorphism has been found in the promoter region for RANTES and association studies have shown this polymorphism to contribute to the development of atopic eczema but not asthma[28].

Although other loci have been linked to atopic eczema, possible candidate genes for these loci have yet to be postulated and identified.

ABNORMAL SKIN BARRIER

Xerosis (dry skin) is a recognized feature of atopic eczema. There are two possible explanations for the dry skin. Either it is a primary defect and part of the atopic syndrome or it is secondary to low-grade eczema, with minimal signs of inflammation.

The dry skin is associated with a defective barrier function, as manifested by increased transepidermal water loss and a low water content of the stratum corneum. This defect in the barrier function of the stratum corneum may lead to the passage of chemicals (e.g. primary irritants) and microorganisms through the stratum corneum and the initiation of an eczematous response. It has been shown that there are alterations in the lipid content of non-eczematous skin in atopic individuals compared to those with non-atopic skin. This alteration in fat content may lead to an alteration in barrier function.

Figure 8 summarizes the possible genetic defects in atopic eczema.

ALLERGENS

Food allergens

It is assumed that atopic eczema is an antigen-dependent disorder. However, the determination of which antigen(s) is the cause of the eczema has so far not been achieved. Parents often implicate food as a cause and it is not infrequent for children to have been given elimination diets by the time they are seen by a dermatologist.

There are reports of some children with atopic eczema who benefit from avoidance of certain foods, and who relapse on re-introduction of these foods. These studies have been double-blind and placebo-controlled. But, in the majority of patients with atopic eczema, it has not been possible to demonstrate any benefit from elimination of particular foods[29].

Elemental diets, consisting of amino acids, carbohydrates, fats, minerals and vitamins, have been tried in patients with atopic eczema. In a controlled study of an elemental diet versus a normal (liquidized diet) in adults with atopic eczema, no difference was shown between the two diets in the clinical features, IgE levels, eosinophil counts and skin biopsies[30]. In a study in children with atopic eczema, an elemental diet was shown to be of some benefit. However, the study was carried out on hospital patients and was not controlled; therefore, some or all of the improvement may have been a placebo effect[31].

Breast-feeding

It has been suggested that breast-feeding is beneficial in preventing atopic eczema. This is thought to be due to the child's lack of exposure to external dietary allergens until later in infancy. However, it is well known that atopic eczema may develop in purely breast-fed children and it has been demonstrated that external dietary antigens can be detected in human breast milk. Thus, breast-fed infants are exposed to dietary antigens and breast-feeding does not totally protect infants from exposure to these antigens. In addition, specific IgE to cow's milk and eggs has been found in infants exclusively breast-fed[32].

Although dietary antigens are present in human breast milk, there may be other benefits from breast-feeding. Secretory IgA is present in breast milk and this may bind to dietary antigens and prevent their absorption. In addition, it has been proposed that other factors present in human breast milk facilitate maturation of the gut and its responses to external antigens[33].

Tests for food allergies

The two types of tests available are 'skin-prick tests' and tests to detect specific IgE antibodies in the serum. The validity of a skin-prick test depends on the presence of antigen-specific IgE on mast cells and elicits a type I hypersensitivity response. Atopic eczema is considered to be a T-cell-mediated, type IV immune response. Thus, the test does not use the pathogenic pathway for inducing eczema and the results are therefore not likely to be relevant. This is found to be so in practice. In routine skin-prick tests for 20 food antigens, usually three to six foods are found to test positive in atopic eczema subjects and, in some instances, the results yield even higher numbers. Yet, when the patient is challenged by the foods giving positive skin-prick tests, only one or two of the foods cause exacerbation of the eczema[34].

Radioallergosorbent tests (RAST) have also been shown to correlate poorly with elimination diets and subsequent challenge for a particular food.

At present, there are no reliable tests for identifying possible foods that may be responsible for inducing or maintaining the eczema. It is possible that, in the majority of individuals with atopic eczema, it is not one or two antigens which cause the eczema but a multitude of foreign antigens, and the fault is in the way the immune system handles these substances. There is a report of finding specific T-cell clones to peanuts in the skin of an infant with atopic eczema. This has been taken to imply that this provides confirmatory evidence that food substances can induce T-cell-specific clones in the skin, thus inducing atopic eczema[35]. However, it has been suggested that the most likely way that infants develop peanut sensitivity is through the application of peanut oil in topical and bath emollients. There are likely to be many T-cell clones to various food substances in blood and skin. Before an etiological role for T-cell clones in the skin to a particular food is accepted, it will have to be shown that removal of this food improves the eczema and that re-introduction induces the eczema.

AEROALLERGENS

Aeroallergens implicated in atopic eczema include house dust mites, molds, pollens and animal dander. The evidence comes partly from clinical data and partly from the results of tests.

Clinical data

House-dust avoidance studies have been shown to benefit some individuals with atopic eczema, but the conduct of these studies under controlled circumstances has proved to be difficult.

There are a small group of patients who have a flare-up of their eczema on areas of skin exposed to the air in the spring and early summer months. This flare-up is thought to be due to pollens released at this time of year. However, this pattern of eczema in the early summer months is uncommon and most patients with atopic eczema benefit from an improvement in their disease condition in summer.

It has also been claimed that aeroallergens that may cause asthma and rhinitis may also cause a flare-up of eczema in atopic individuals when the allergen is administered intranasally or by bronchial inhalation[35]. Yet this response does not occur in all patients with atopic eczema and it is said only to occur in subjects with IgE antibodies to the particular allergen used for challenge.

Patch tests

The so-called atopy patch test has been used to try to predict whether patients are sensitive to a particular aeroallergen. If the patch test is positive, yielding an eczematous response, this implies that the aeroallergen can induce atopic eczema in the individual, although, in this instance, the aeroallergen is acting as a contact allergen. However, the conditions under which the allergen is tested are not the same as those in which the allergen may come into contact with the skin in an atopic patient. In the early studies on house dust mites, positive reactions were only obtained after Sell-o-tape stripping of the stratum corneum and not with a normal intact skin barrier. The results, therefore, imply that house dust mites cannot induce eczema in patients with an intact stratum corneum.

The most recent study on patch tests to aeroallergens in atopic individuals did not find a correlation between the clinical features and patch test results, and concluded that, at present, there was no indication for patch tests in the management of atopic eczema[36].

AUTOANTIGENS

As in most chronic inflammatory disorders, the possible role of autoantigens in maintaining the disease, even if not initiating it, has been proposed for atopic eczema. Studies have shown that human dander can trigger hypersensitivity responses, and this suggests an IgE-mediated response. IgE antibodies have been reported against human proteins. Although attempts have been made to clone and identify the autoantigens in IgE complexes, so far no specific antigen has been identified.

BACTERIA

Bacteria on the surface of the skin have been implicated in the etiology of atopic eczema for over 100 years. Gram-positive cocci were the organisms considered to be responsible for the eczema and it was said that, if *Staphylococci* were brought into contact with slightly irritated skin, eczema could be induced after 24 h. *Streptococci* were also implicated in eczema and streptococcal vaccines were tried as a treatment. More recently, discussion on the role of *Staphylococci* in atopic eczema has been revived. *Staphylococcus aureus* is found in 100% of acute exudative lesions of atopic eczema, in approximately 90% of chronic lesions, and in 65% of clinically normal unaffected skin of individuals with atopic eczema[37]. *S.aureus* is found on the skin in less than 5% of normal non-atopic individuals. However, the important question is whether the staphylococcal organisms play a role in the pathogenesis of the eczema or whether the atopic skin simply provides a good environment, which encourages colonization by the organism. The presence of the organisms may be secondary to the abnormality of the atopic skin, both involved and uninvolved.

There are a number of mechanisms by which *S. aureus* organisms may induce the eczematous process. It has been shown that, in a significant proportion of individuals with atopic eczema, there is a high incidence of specific IgE antibodies to *S. aureus*.

IgE antibodies are more common in patients with severe and chronic eczematous lesions[38]. It is thought that the continual scratching in chronic atopic eczema allows greater colonization by *S. aureus* because of the damaged barrier caused by scratching. It has been suggested that the staphylo-coccal IgE antibodies may be pathogenic and may play a role in an inflammatory reaction. Conversely, the antibodies may be of a secondary nature and may not be important to the pathogenesis of eczema.

S.aureus may also induce eczema by the same pathway as other antigens, e.g. food and aeroallergens, by binding to IgE receptors on antigen-presenting cells in the skin and activating specific T-cells (Figure 9).

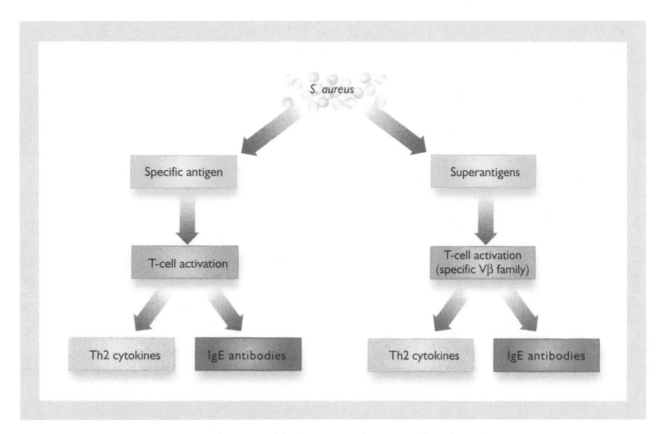

Figure 9 *S. aureus* may activate T-cell in atopic eczema, either by a superantigen or specific antigen effect

More recently, superantigens secreted by *S. aureus* organisms have been implicated in the pathogenesis. Superantigens induce activation of T-cells and macrophages. In addition, they up-regulate CLA expression on lymphocytes, thus enabling them to target the skin. They also induce a T-cell receptor V family expansion. This results in the production of a large number of activated T-cells in the skin in a short space of time, and these can induce an inflammatory reaction, as seen in eczema (Figure 9). Superantigens have also been shown to increase the synthesis of allergen-specific IgE antibodies, and these in turn increase the severity of the eczema. In support of this hypothesis, it has been shown that the application of staphylococcal enterotoxin B to the uninvolved skin of atopic subjects induces eczema[39] (Figure 10).

The colonization of the skin by *S.aureus* may depend on the increased adherence of the organism in atopic skin. Adherence of the bacteria to epithelial cells is the initial step in the pathogenesis of many infections. It has been shown that *S.aureus* has a much greater degree of adherence to corneocytes affected by atopic eczema than those from normal individuals and those with other inflammatory skin conditions such as psoriasis[37]. The adhesins that enable *S.aureus* to bind to the skin are thought to be extracellular matrix components, including fibronectin. Interestingly, in binding studies of *S.aureus* to the skin, it was shown that, in skin lesions with a Th2 inflammatory response compared to a Th1 response, bacterial binding was greater in the Th2-mediated inflammation. This may be due to fibronectin induction by IL-4 (Figure 11).

The innate immune system has recently been described and implicated in atopic eczema. This system in the skin is triggered by a number of receptors for microbial components. The best-defined receptors are Toll-like receptors (TLRs). These receptors on epithelial cells, when activated, can induce the release of antimicrobial peptides, which have been termed human -defensins (HBDs) and cathelicidins. These peptides can attract T-cells, immature dendritic cells and neutrophils, and are intended to provide a protective response against invading bacteria. It has recently been shown in patients with atopic eczema that there are low levels of two antimicrobial peptides, the human defensin, HBD-2 and the cathelicidin, LL-37[40]. Both these peptides are concerned with controlling the growth of *S.aureus* on the skin. It has also been shown that the cytokines IL-4 and IL-13, which are Th2 cytokines and are increased in eczema, can inhibit the induction of antimicrobial peptides HBD-2 and LL-37. Thus, it has been implied that the low levels of these two antimicrobial peptides may be a secondary event in atopic eczema and not a primary one. This further implies that *S.aureus* colonization of skin in patients with atopic eczema is not a primary initiating cause of atopic eczema. An additional observation that argues against a primary role for *S.aureus* in atopic eczema is the fact that topical steroids and tacrolimus will heal the eczematous process, and the staphylococcal colonization, present before treatment, will disappear with treatment. Thus, colonization with *S. aureus* would appear to be dependent on the existing eczematous process.

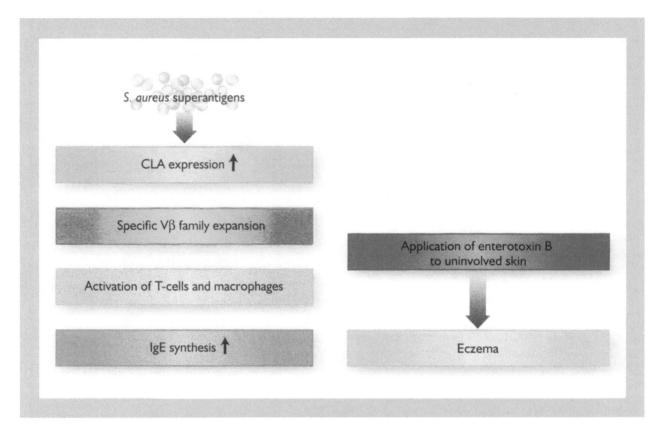

Figure 10 Effects of superantigens, which may induce atopic eczema. CLA, cutaneous lymphocyte antigen; V , part of the T-cell receptor

FUNGI

A number of fungi that are normal inhabitants of the skin, *Malassezia furfur* and *Candida albicans,* may play some part in the pathogenesis of atopic eczema. If these organisms penetrate the skin, for example when the skin barrier is weakened or when the skin barrier is broken due to scratching, they can induce Th1- or Th2-dependent immune responses. Most normal individuals will show a cell-mediated response to *C.albicans*. However, in atopics, there is often a type 1 hypersensitivity response with redness, itching, and an urticarial reaction. Although, *M.furfur* and *C.albicans* are not likely to have a primary role in atopic eczema, they may possibly have an aggravating effect.

ENVIRONMENTAL POLLUTION

There has been an increase in the incidence of atopic eczema over the last 50 years. Although there is a strong genetic component to the disease, environmental factors also appear to play a role. Air pollutants have been suspected of playing a possible role in this increased incidence. They would act as non-specific irritants rather than allergens, but they also appear to have an immunomodulating effect, i.e. they have been shown to enhance IgE formation in animals.

It should also be mentioned that some forms of air pollution have decreased in the last 50 years. The burning of coal, which was associated with smog and high sulfur content in the atmosphere, has decreased considerably. The pollution that has increased is caused by the oxides of nitrogen and sulfur and the photochemical oxidants such as ozone. Most of the pollutants are from the petrochemicals used in the automobile industry. There appears to be some correlation between increasing levels of sulfur dioxide and oxides of nitrogen and atopic eczema[41]. This is true for hay fever and, to a lesser extent, for asthma. Smoking during pregnancy has also been found to be a risk factor.

HYGIENE HYPOTHESIS

One of the theories suggested to account for the increase in atopic disorders over the last few decades has been the so-called 'hygiene hypothesis'. The hypothesis is that children born in the latter half of the twentieth century have less bacterial and viral infection in early life compared to children born in the first half of the century. This has resulted in the immune response being Th2-skewed. Infections by bacteria and viruses induce a Th1 response and these infections in early life will convert the infant to a Th1 response when exposed to allergens. Lack of exposure to bacteria and viruses and control of infections with

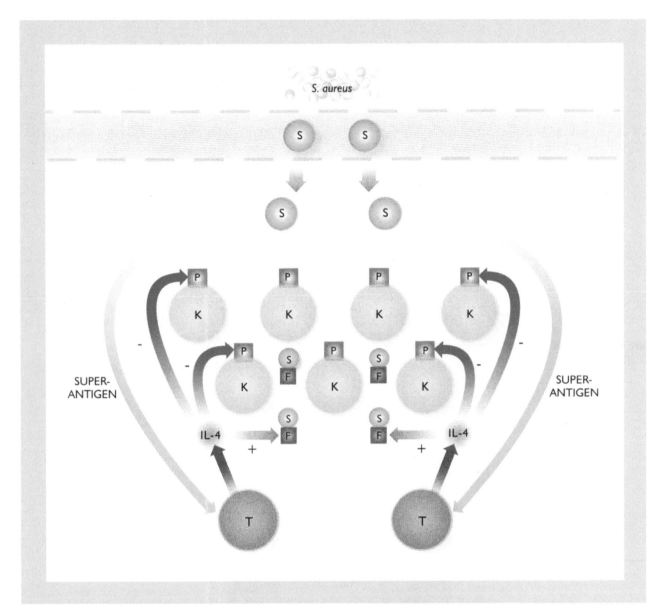

Figure 11 Antimicrobial peptides in the innate immune system are down-regulated in atopic eczema. This may be due to IL-4 produced by activated T-cells. In addition, IL-4 induces fibronectin, which enhances adherence of *S.aureus,* an essential step in colonization of the skin in the pathogenesis of infections. S, *S.aureus;* K, keratinocyte; T, T-cell; F, fibronectin; P, innate immune system peptide

antibiotics will delay the conversion of the immune system to a Th1 response and the Th2 response is maintained for a longer time. Therefore, when the subject is exposed to potential allergens, a Th2 or 'allergic' response results.

Support for this hygiene hypothesis comes from a study in Sweden comparing the children of families with an anthroposophic lifestyle and a control group[42]. Anthroposophy originates from a Greek word and means 'wisdom about man'. Anthroposophy, as a way of life, was founded in the twentieth century by Rudolph Steiner and has been applied to art, architecture, agriculture and medicine. In anthroposophic medicine, the use of antibiotics, antipyretics, and vaccinations is restricted. Vaccinations are usually only given against polio and tetanus and then later in life than usually recommended. In addition, children follow-ing the anthroposophic way of life consume local foods produced according to biodynamic principles. Vegetables preserved by spontaneous fermentation are a common dietary element and probably contain live lactobacilli, which are probiotics. In the study, 295 children following the anthroposophic lifestyle were compared to 380 controls. There was a significant lower incidence of atopy in children following the anthroposophic lifestyle and this incidence strongly correlated with the strictness of the lifestyle features[42].

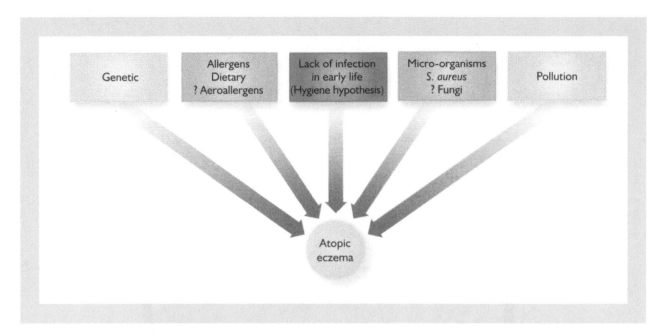

Figure 12 Summary of etiological factors in atopic eczema

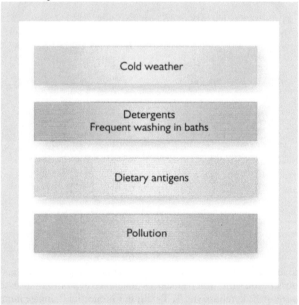

Figure 13 Possible triggers for atopic eczema

PHARMACOLOGICAL AND VASCULAR ABNORMALITIES

There are a number of abnormalities that relate to the control of small blood vessels in atopic eczema. It has long been known that patients report pallor of the skin, and hypersensitivity to cold with vasoconstriction and low finger temperature. White dermographism has been attributed to an increase in catecholamines in the nerve endings in atopic skin. Yet it has been reported that there is a decrease of adrenergic nerve fibers in atopic skin lesions. Thus, the vasoconstriction may be caused by increased sensitivity to catecholamines or perhaps there is another pharmacological mediator causing the vasoconstriction. There is a delayed blanch to acetylcholine. The method by which these abnormalities relate to the development of atopic eczema is not yet known. It is possible they represent an abnormal neuropeptide profile in atopics.

EMOTIONAL FACTORS

There is no doubt that emotional stress can make atopic disease worse. This effect could be mediated by the immune system, hormones or neuropeptides. It is a relatively unexplored field.

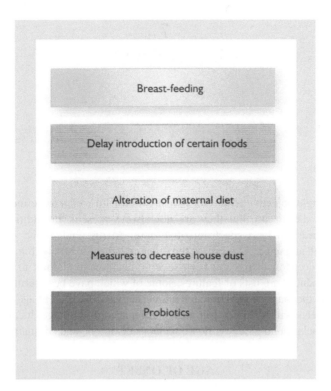

Figure 14 Practical measures based on etiological factors that may be of benefit in management

NEUROPEPTIDES

Peptides are released by nerve endings in tissue. This is a relatively under-researched area, but neuro-peptides are biologically active substances and may well influence immune responses. Thickening of nerve fibers has been described in the skin, and related to continual scratching. However, whether this is the cause is not proven. Neuropeptides may also be involved in the intense pruritus associated with atopic eczema.

SUMMARY

The definite etiological factor is genetic. Allergens, or in other words, foreign proteins, either dietary or aeroallergens, probably play a role and the other possible contributory factors include micro-organisms, pollution and the 'hygiene hypothesis' (Figure 12).

Possible triggers (Figure 13) and helpful measures (Figure 14) are discussed in more detail in the chapter on 'Management'.

7
Clinical features

At the present time, there is no single objective feature or investigation with which to define atopic eczema. There are certain clinical features characteristic of the disease but they are not always present. In addition, as in many disorders with a multifactorial etiology, there appears to be a spectrum of disease. At one end of the spectrum are patients with many recognized features associated with atopic eczema, but, at the other end, are patients with mild disease and only one or two of these features. Over the last two decades, there have been several meetings to attempt to define the clinical state of atopic eczema, but the best outcomes produced are lists of features, some of which have been termed major and other minor[3,43]. The problem is further complicated by the fact that the clinical features can vary in different age groups.

In this chapter, the clinical aspects will be divided in presentation according to age, localized sites of atopic skin disease, associated skin disorders with a background of atopy, non-cutaneous disorders, and stigmata associated with atopic eczema.

AGE OF ONSET

Atopic eczema may present at any age but is essentially a childhood disorder. The most common age of onset is between 2 and 6 months. In the majority, the eczema will present before the age of 2 years.

SEX

Males and females appear to be equally affected.

CLINICAL FEATURES OF ECZEMA PER SE

Before considering the specific features of atopic eczema, it should be appreciated that there are other clinical patterns of eczema. Many features are common to all these patterns of eczema, depending on the severity of the eczematous process. In mild forms, the skin is red and scaly (Figure 15); in the severe forms (subacute eczema), the skin may be 'edematous', due to tissue fluid, and, on the surface, there is crusting. Crusts represent the breaking down of the epidermis, with serum seeping from the surface but coagulating to form a yellow dried surface (Figures 16 and 17). In the most severe forms (acute eczema), the stratum corneum is lost and a weeping moist surface is evident (Figure 18).

In the chronic forms of eczema, there may be a thickened stratum corneum (hyperkeratosis), which often splits, forming fissures (Figure 19), or the whole of the skin is thickened. This latter feature is typical of atopic eczema and is often referred to as lichenification (Figure 20). This word is derived from the term 'lichen', a plant which grows on rocks, causing a thickened surface. Lichenification is said to occur in atopics due to continual scratching. However, there is probably an underlying constitutional factor in atopics that allows this   thickening to develop, since there are many other skin disorders associated with pruritus and continual scratching in which lichenification does not occur.

AGE-RELATED FEATURES

Infants

The eczema usually first appears on the face and is seen as red patches, which may or may not be scaly (Figures 21–23). If the condition is acute, weeping and crusting will be seen (Figures 24 and 25). Any part of the face may be affected.

Involvement may also be seen on the trunk (Figures 26 and 27) and limbs (Figures 28–34). In this age group, it presents as red scaly patches. Occasionally, the patches may coalesce and the eruption is confluent (Figures 28 and 29). If the inflammation is severe, then the patches may form crusts and weep. The crusts are characteristically golden, since they are formed of a mixture of serum and keratin. Occasionally, the patches are red and raised and urticarial in appearance, and this

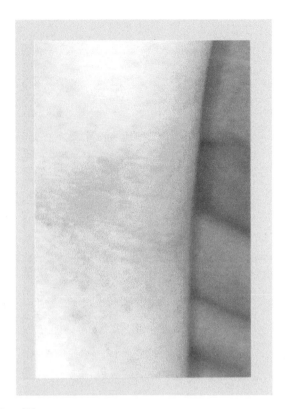

Figure 15 Redness and minimal scaling in mild eczema

can subsequently progress to scaling, crusting or weeping, depending on the severity of the inflammation. Although atopic eczema classically involves the flexures of the knees and elbows, in infants the involvement is frequently on the extensor surfaces of the limbs when the disease first presents (Figures 28, 30–32).

The scalp may be involved and, in its mildest form, will present as scaling (dandruff). In the more acute stage, crusted areas may be present.

Itching is a feature of atopic eczema and infants will scratch involuntarily and thus the lesions are often excoriated, presenting as scabs (Figures 33 and 34), some of which may have a linear conformity. Excoriating the skin may also give rise to secondary bacterial infection. This is usually due to *Staphylococcus aureus* but -hemolytic streptococcal infections may also occur. In infection with S. *aureus,* the lesions often develop golden crusts and/or weeping (Figure 35). It may be difficult to distinguish between acute weeping eczema (not infected) and secondarily infected eczema (Figure 36). Pustules are occasionally seen, making the diagnosis of secondary infection easier (Figure 36). In secondary infection with streptococci, erythema and edema of the skin surrounding the eczematous lesions are present.

Childhood, age 2±12 years

The common sites of atopic eczema in this age group are the flexures of the knees (Figure 37) and elbows (Figures 38 and 39) (hence the term flexural eczema). Other common sites are the wrists (Figure 40), ankles (Figure 41), neck, gluteal folds (Figure 42) and face. However, in severe disease, the involvement extends beyond these sites and may involve the trunk and large areas of the limbs (Figures 43–45). Occasionally, the eczema may involve the extensor surfaces of the knees (Figure 31) and elbows, the so-called 'reverse pattern eczema'. This is thought to be a more persistent form of the disease and carries a poorer prognosis.

The lesions appear as red scaly areas (Figures 37 and 42), or crusting and weeping ones in the acute stages and thickened (lichenified) skin, particularly on the limbs, in the chronic phase (Figures 44 and 45). The lichenified patches are red or sometimes pale. The surface may be scaly and there is increased linearity of the skin surface markings. Excoriations (Figures 39, 44 and 45) are common and secondary infection, as seen in infants, may also occur (Figure 46).

Lichenified eczema, particularly on the limbs, is more common in Asians and black people (Figures 47 and 48) and is more resistant to treatment.

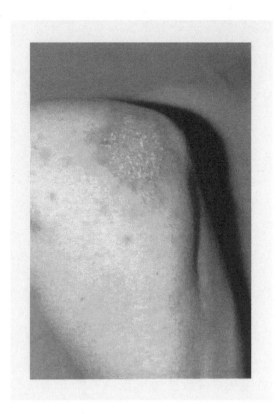

Figure 16 Subacute eczema with yellowish crusts

Adolescents and adults

During childhood, atopic eczema usually improves and goes into remission in the majority of individuals. In a small proportion, usually less than 10%, the eczema continues into adulthood. In addition, in some individuals who had childhood eczema, the disease may have gone into remission for several years but recurs in adult life, often associated with stress. Very occasionally, atopic eczema may present for the first time in adult life. Whether this is a true primary presentation or whether patients have no recollection of eczema in childhood is debatable.

In adults, lichenified patches on the flexures of the knees and elbows (Figures 49–52) may occur, as in children. Involvement of the face (Figures 53–55), particularly around the eyes, is another presentation. The eyelids and surrounding skin are red, swollen and scaly (Figures 53 and 54). Patches or confluent involvement on the neck also occur (Figures 56 and 57). Occasionally in severe disease,   the eczema is generalized and the skin is red, scaly and lichenified all over. This is sometimes referred to as erythroderma (Figure 58).

NON-AGE-RELATED FEATURES

Symmetry

As with other forms of endogenous skin disease, atopic eczema tends to be a symmetrical eruption (Figures 31, 37–40, 43, 49, 52). It is usual for all the lesions to show similar clinical features at one time, i.e. if the lesions are acute with weeping and crusting, then these lesions are found in a symmetrical pattern. If the lesions are asymmetrical, then this may imply secondary bacterial infection of the eczema. The reasons for symmetry of skin lesions in eczema or in other diseases, e.g. psoriasis, are as yet unknown. One possibility is that receptors in the endothelium of cutaneous vessels have developed symmetrically, as has the human body. In eczema and psoriasis, the rash is dependent on inflammatory cells coming into the skin via specialized receptors.

Altered pigmentation

Inflammation in the skin may either stimulate or suppress melanocyte function. Thus, the skin at the sites of the eczema may either become darker (Figures 59 and 60) or paler (Figures 61 and 62). The pigmentary changes often become more apparent

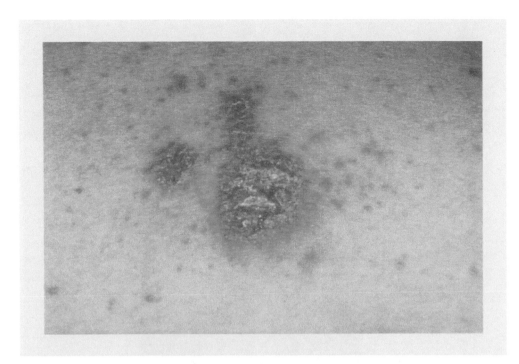

Figure 17 Subacute eczema with crusts and some erosions

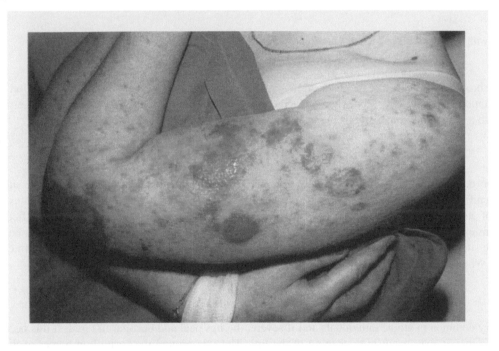

Figure 18 Loss of surface of the skin with a weeping surface in acute eczema

after the eczema has cleared. Both the hypo- and hyperpigmentation will resolve and the skin return to its normal color, although it may take many months.

Hypo- and hyperpigmentary changes are more apparent in dark-skinned and particularly black individuals, as it seems their melanocytes are more susceptible to inflammatory changes.

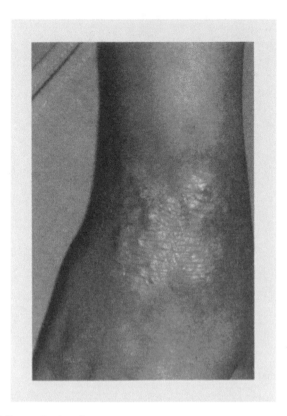

Figure 19 Soles with hyperkeratosis and fissures in chronic eczema

Reticulate pigmentation on the neck

In adults with chronic atopic eczema, the neck often shows a reticulate pattern of increased pigmentation (Figure 63). This type of pigmentation is usually only seen when the acute inflammatory component of the eczema has been suppressed. If the eczema goes into a long remission, then this pigmentation will slowly improve.

ATOPIC ECZEMA AT SPECIFIC SITES

Occasionally, eczema may occur at specific sites, with or without involvement at the more characteristic sites. If the classical lesions of lichenified eczema in the flexures are present, then the eczema at these other specific sites is accepted as a manifestation of atopic eczema. However, if the eczema is only present at specific sites, it is more difficult to accept these lesions as a manifestation of atopic disease. The sites in question are the lips, soles, and the nipples and areolae on the breasts. Eczema at these sites is thought to be a manifestation of atopic eczema because it is commonly seen with classical lesions of atopic eczema. When it occurs solely at these sites, there is a strong personal or family history of atopy.

LipsÐcheilitis

Dry lips are very common in atopic individuals and if severe, the lips peel and become fissured. If this becomes chronic, the associated inflammation may result in thickening of the lips. The skin around the vermillion border of the lip may also be affected and this presents as redness and scaling (Figure 64). It is often aggravated and becomes persistent when the child develops the habit of 'lip licking' to try and moisten the dry sore lips. The problem is also worse in the cold weather when the low temperatures exacerbate the dryness of the lips. In dark-skinned individuals, there is often associated hyperpigmenta-tion around the lips that may be the feature that prompts the patient or their parents to seek medical advice.

Peri-auricular eczema

Redness, scaling and fissuring at the base of (Figure 65) and behind (Figure 66) the pinna is another common feature of atopic eczema. It may or may not be associated with eczema at other sites.

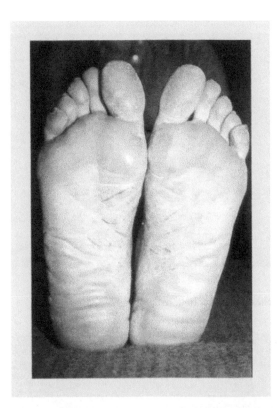

Figure 20 Lichenification and thickened plaques, a feature of atopic eczema which is common in black people

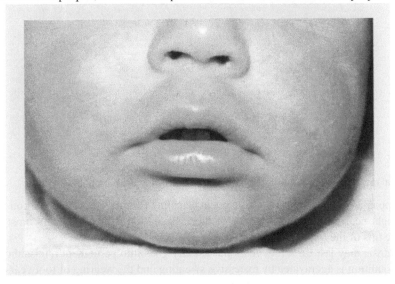

Figure 21 Red, slightly scaly cheeks, upper lip, and chin in early atopic eczema

Breast eczema

Eczema manifested by itching, crusting and scaling on the areola and nipples is not uncommon. Fortunately, it is usually bilateral. If it is unilateral, a diagnosis of Paget's disease has to be considered. This pattern may be the only feature of atopic eczema in young female adults.

Juvenile plantar dermatosis

This is a distinct clinical entity in which there is involvement on the distal half of the sole and plantar surface of the toes (Figure 67). It is most commonly seen between the ages of 8 and 16 years, and is slightly more common in males.

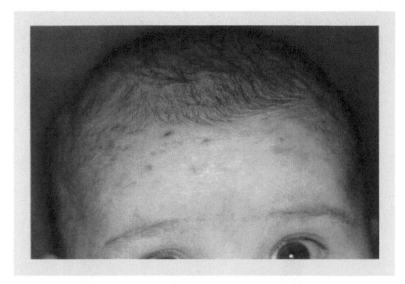

Figure 22 Mild atopic eczema on the forehead with excoriations

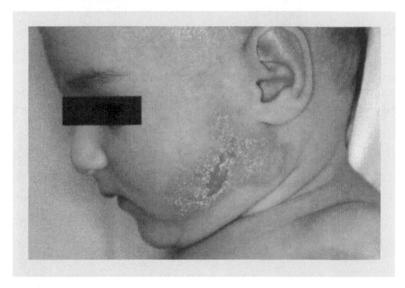

Figure 23 More severe facial involvement in atopic eczema. Scaling and crusting are present

The skin has a shiny appearance with superficial fissures and scaling (Figure 67). The condition has been termed the 'shiny foot' syndrome. The weight-bearing areas on the balls of the feet and toe pads are usually most severely affected. Similar lesions may appear on the tips of the fingers.

Juvenile plantar dermatosis may last for a few years but usually goes into permanent remission during adolescence. It has been suggested that the condition is aggravated by excessive sweating and the wearing of footwear made from plastic. Leather and/or fabric shoes are thought to be more appropriate. Cotton socks should also be recommended.

Atopic hand eczema

Involvement is mainly on the dorsal surface of the fingers and hands (Figure 68), which is the opposite of pompholyx eczema, which affects the palms and sides of the fingers. Involvement of the back of the hands in atopic eczema is common in children and may continue into adulthood or recur in adult life after a long remission at these sites. The lesions are red lichenified scaly patches (Figure 69), often with fissures (Figure 70), particularly over the joints where the skin is stretched when the fingers are flexed. If the skin proximal to the nail, where the nail matrix is sited, is involved, then nail plate abnormalities may be seen. These consist of ridging and pits in the nail.

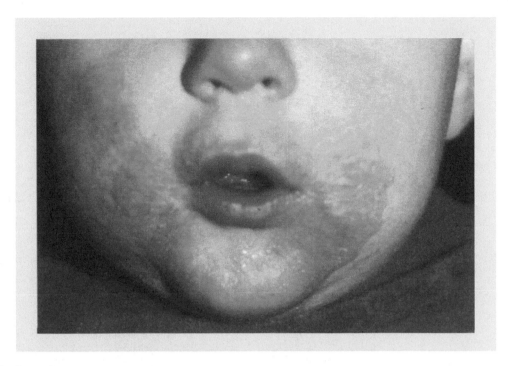

Figure 24 Crusting in atopic eczema

OTHER ECZEMATOUS SKIN DISORDERS IN ATOPIC INDIVIDUALS

Pityriasis alba

Pityriasis means scaly and alba means white. Pityriasis alba is usually seen in children and young adolescents. It occurs mostly on the cheeks and presents as hypopigmented (not depigmented) areas with an ill-defined edge (Figure 71). Sometimes, there is a preceding history of mild scaling and even redness prior to the pale patches appearing.

Pityriasis alba is most commonly seen in dark-skinned children, since there is a sharper contrast between the affected and unaffected skin. In Caucasian children, pityriasis alba often presents after they have been on holiday in the sun. The affected areas fail to tan, whereas the unaffected areas tan normally. It is likely that pityriasis alba is a low-grade eczema, which interferes with pigment production. If the affected areas are treated as for eczema, the normal pigmentation usually returns after 2–3 months.

A similar condition to pityriasis alba on the face in children is seen on the outer arms in young adult females. It usually presents after the individual has been on holiday in a sunny climate and has failed to tan in sites where they have low-grade eczema. The condition can be prevented by applying a topical steroid ointment for 2 weeks before going in the sun.

Discoid papular eczema

In this condition, scaly follicular papules occur in a discoid pattern. These lesions, which may occur on the limbs (Figure 72) or trunk, may be solitary or multiple and symmetrical.

Lichen simplex

The term implies thickening of the skin in a localized patch. Essentially, it is a localized patch of lichen-ification (Figure 73) and is most commonly seen on the outer lower legs in men and back of the neck in females. It is due to a habit of continuously excoriating one area. It tends to be a very persistent problem.

Prurigo nodularis

The term prurigo means 'itchy' and nodularis refers to firm lumps in the skin. The condition is most commonly seen in middle-aged females. There is often an underlying psychological problem. The lesions are seen most commonly on the extensor surfaces of the limbs (Figure 74), since these are the areas that are most accessible for scratching. The patient

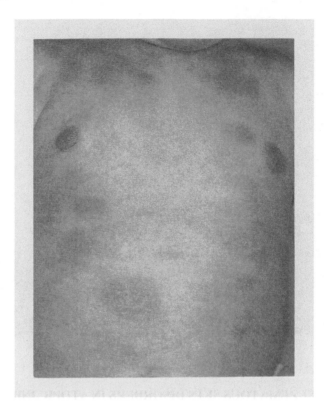

Figure 25 Crusting in severe atopic eczema

develops a habit of picking and excoriating the lesions, resulting in local lichenification. Approximately three-quarters of patients have a past history of atopic eczema.

NON-ECZEMATOUS CUTANEOUS FEATURES OF ATOPY

Xeroderma

Xeroderma means dry skin and is derived from the Greek word *xeros* meaning dry. Patients with atopic eczema or a past history often complain that their skin is dry and/or slightly flaky. In addition, individuals who have never had eczema but who have a dry skin often have a family history of atopic disease or a personal history of asthma and hay fever.

Dryness is essentially an abnormal shedding of the stratum corneum/keratin layer (the skin barrier). It is thought that the bonding of the corneocytes is impaired, leading to increased loss of keratin. Keratin bonding is temperature-dependent. The lower the temperature, the less the bonding and thus the drier the skin. Atopic subjects often complain that their skin is drier and cracks more easily in the winter months.

The decreased keratin bonding and associated loss of skin barrier function are considered to be one of the essential defects in atopic eczema.

Keratosis pilaris

Keratosis pilaris is caused by excess keratin formation, which plugs the orifice of the hair follicle. It presents as rough papules and the most common sites are the upper and outer arms (Figure 75). It is most commonly seen in young adults and there is a sexual predilection for females. It may also occur on the front of the thighs, buttocks and upper back. In some instances, erythema surrounds the keratotic follicular papule. The condition is worse in the winter months and improves in warm climates. There is a strong association with atopy.

Increased linearity on the palms and soles

This is associated with dry skin and is another feature of the impaired keratin-bonding characteristic of atopics (Figure 76).

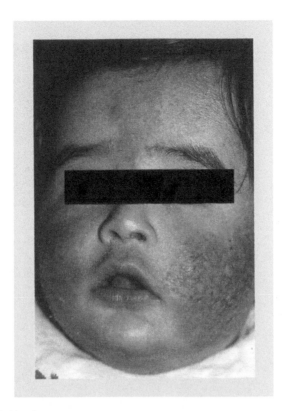

Figure 26 Patches of atopic eczema on the trunk

Micropapular eruption on the trunk in black people

In atopic black children, a distinct micropapular eruption is seen on the trunk, particularly the abdomen. This eruption is not an eczematous process and is not itchy. It tends to disappear with age and is not a feature in adult atopic subjects.

Dennie-Morgan infraorbital fold

This is defined as two lines, with a fold of skin in between, and is found below the lower eyelid (Figure 77). Normal individuals tend to have one or no lines under the eyes. Although there is a definite association with atopic disease, it is not as strong as other features described above.

Skin pallor

Patients with atopic eczema often have a pale complexion, associated with vasoconstriction of the superficial cutaneous blood vessels. This may be due to increased sensitivity to cold, with resulting vasoconstriction. Atopics tend to have cold hands, another feature of cold sensitivity.

White dermographism

If an eczematous area in an atopic individual is subjected to linear pressure with a blunt instrument, a white line will appear after approximately 30 s and this stays white for a few moments (Figure 78).

OTHER DISORDERS ASSOCIATED WITH ATOPIC ECZEMA

Asthma

Asthma is one of the three disorders that constitute the atopic triad: asthma, eczema and hay fever. Approximately 25–30% of patients with atopic eczema will develop asthma at some stage of their life. In half of these, allergic rhinitis also occurs. The asthma commences before the age of 5 in one-third of those that develop the condition.

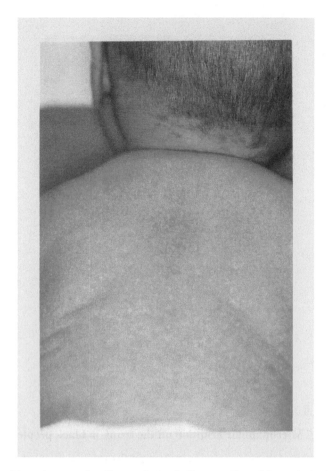

Figure 27 Confluent atopic eczema with erythema and scaling on the back. Some scaling of the scalp is also present

Allergic rhinitis (hay fever)

This will subsequently occur in 50% of patients with atopic eczema and usually begins between the ages of 10 and 30, which is considerably later than atopic eczema. Allergic rhinitis is often associated with allergic conjunctivitis (Figure 79) to varying degrees. At times, the nasal symptoms predominate, whilst in others the conjunctivitis is the major symptom.

Approximately one-third of patients with atopic eczema will not develop either asthma or allergic rhinitis, while 10% will have all three disorders. These findings suggest both common and specific etiological factors for the development of these three atopic disorders.

Urticaria and migraine

Although migraine and urticaria are not considered to be part of the atopic state, there does appear to be an increased incidence in so-called atopic individuals. Migraine and urticaria may have specific external triggers, as do the classical atopic disorders. However, the exact pathogenetic mechanisms have not been elucidated for migraine, urticaria and atopic disorders, and thus there is speculation whether there could be a common predisposing factor to these diseases.

Atopic keratoconjunctivitis

This is distinct from the 'allergic' conjunctivitis that occurs with rhinitis. In kerotoconjunctivitis, the eyelids are lichenified, crusted and scaly and the conjunctiva is hyperemic (Figure 80). There may be associated keratitis, and repeated attacks may lead to scarring and vascularization of the cornea, with eventual loss of sight.

Keratoconus

This is progressive bulging of the cornea, which produces visual defects (Figure 81). The cause is unknown but it is more common in atopic subjects.

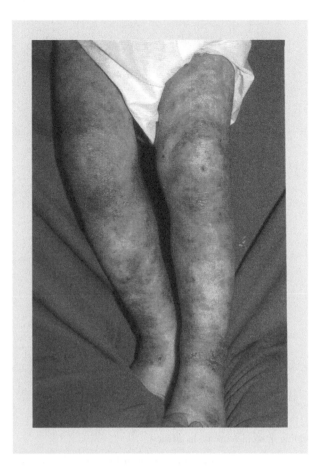

Figure 28 Extensive involvement on the extensor surface of the legs in an infant

Ichthyosis vulgaris

Ichthyosis vulgaris is a distinct clinical entity. There is a reported increased incidence in individuals with atopic eczema compared to normal subjects[44]. Clinically, it presents as dry scaly skin and may be confused with general dry skin, which is a feature of atopic eczema itself. Ichthyosis vulgaris is most pronounced on the lower legs and, in its mildest form, it may be the only site affected. In its more severe forms, the involvement is extensive, although there is sparing of the flexures of the limbs (Figure 82). Both ichthyosis vulgaris and the xeroderma of atopic eczema improve in the warm weather and deteriorate in cold climates. Both conditions are defects in keratin bonding, which is temperature-dependent.

INFECTIONS

There is an increased incidence and severity of infections associated with certain bacteria, viruses and fungal microorganisms. There are two possible explanations for this observation: first, a defect in the barrier function of the stratum corneum and, second, an altered immune response to certain microorganisms.

Bacterial infection

Staphylococcal infections are common in patients with atopic eczema. There appear to be two clinical patterns. In the first, localized patches of eczema become infected with *S.aureus;* this infection responds well to antibacterial treatment. In the second, there seems to be an inability of the subject to deal with the organism and this manifests as recurrent infection.

Staphylococcal infection is suggested by weeping and crusting of the lesions. The crusts are often yellow and small blisters may be seen at the periphery (Figure 36). In the second pattern of infection, there is frequently weeping and crusting on the face (Figure 46) and particularly around the eyes and ears. There is often a good response to oral and topical antibiotics but a rapid relapse when treatment is discontinued. Even treatment of the staphylococcal carrier sites seems unable to prevent relapse. Indefinite antibacterial measures may be required.

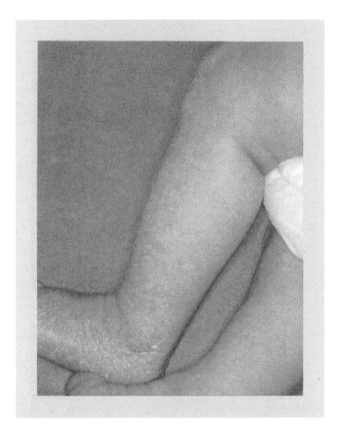

Figure 29 Confluent erythema and scaling in atopic eczema in infancy

Cutaneous fungal infections

Infections of the nails and skin with *Trichophyton rubrum* have been reported to be increased in atopic eczema. The sites of involvement are particularly the hands and feet. Interestingly, there have been reports of an increased incidence of *Trichophyton rubrum* infection of nails in psoriasis.

Pityrosporum oribiculare is a saprophytic yeast, which is found on normal skin but, under certain conditions, can be pathogenic. In atopic individuals, *P. orbiculare* has been associated with an acute flare of eczema on the head, neck and shoulders.

Viral infections

There is a slightly increased incidence in atopic patients of herpes simplex 1 and 2, viral warts (Figure 68) and molluscum contagiosum (Figure 83) compared to non-atopic individuals of the same age. It is important to try to avoid topical corticosteroid preparations at the sites of these viral infections, as particularly herpes simplex and mollusca lesions tend to spread if these preparations are used at the site of the infection. This can present a problem in management since frequently the mollusca lesions occur at sites of atopic eczema.

Eczema herpeticum and eczema vaccinatum

Herpes simplex and vaccinia viruses and rarely Coxsackie A16 can cause a widespread acute cutaneous eruption in atopic individuals, referred to as eczema herpeticum (herpes simplex) and eczema vaccinatum (vaccinia infection). With the eradication of smallpox, world-wide vaccination against smallpox with vaccina virus has been discontinued. However, the smallpox virus is still found in some experimental laboratories and, with the threat of bioterrorism using the virus, mass vaccination may be reintroduced.

Clinically, it is not possible to distinguish between eczema herpeticum and eczema vaccinatum. The eruption begins as an acute blistering eruption, particularly on the face (Figures 84 and 85) and neck, with a few lesions elsewhere on the trunk and limbs. The blisters quickly break and give rise to crusted ulcerated lesions (Figures 85 and 86), which often become secondarily infected with *S.aureus.*

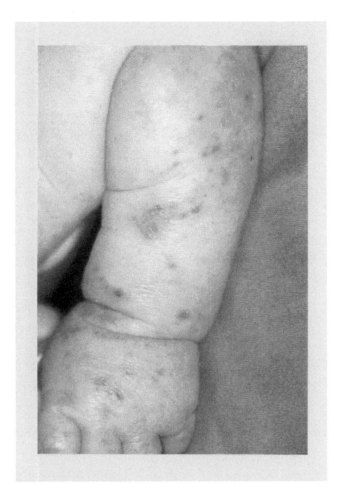

Figure 30 Atopic eczema on the extensor surface of the arms of an infant

Eczema herpeticum has a high morbidity and occasionally, if untreated, may prove fatal if the internal organs are involved. Meningoencephalitis, pneumonitis, hepatitis and colitis have all been reported. Herpetic infections of the eye (keratoconjunctivitis) are common in eczema herpeticum.

Fortunately, with the advent of effective antiviral drugs (aciclovir, famciclovir) against herpes simplex virus, eczema herpeticum now has a better prognosis. If the disease is suspected on clinical grounds, it is important to start antiviral treatment immediately and not wait for laboratory confirmation of the infection. It is also advisable to commence antibacterial therapy at the same time because of possible secondary infection with *S. aureus*.

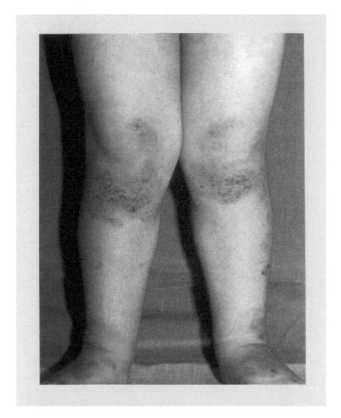

Figure 31 Extensor surface involvement on the knees in an infant. Crusting and excoriations are present

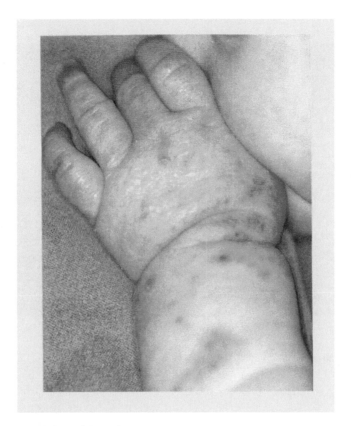

Figure 32 Back of the hand and arm in an infant with atopic eczema

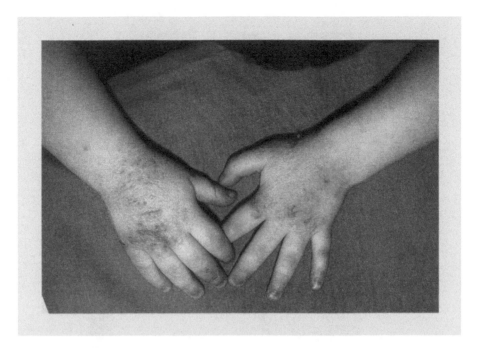

Figure 33 Eczema showing excoriations

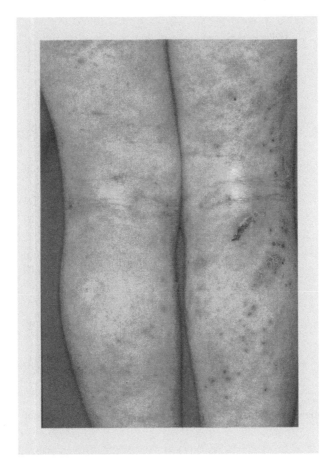

Figure 34 Excoriations and crusting in infantile atopic eczema

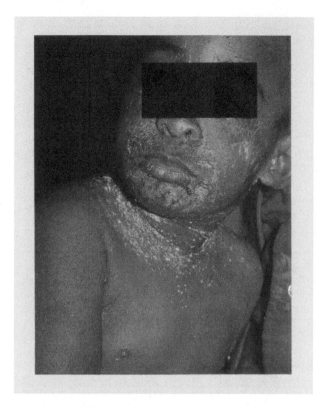

Figure 35 Secondarily infected eczema with *S.aureus*. Crusting and superficial erosions are present

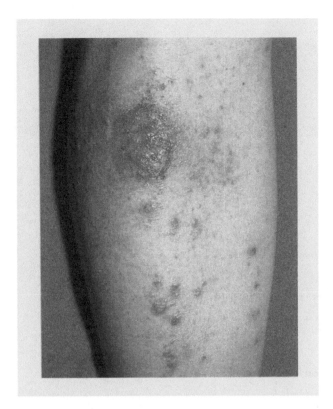

Figure 36 Secondarily infected eczema, with weeping surface and satellite papules, vesicles and papules

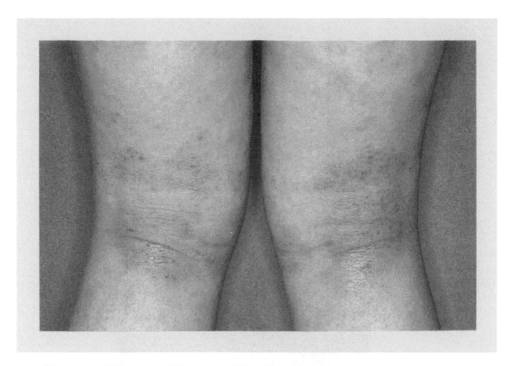

Figure 37 Involvement of the popliteal fossae, one of the common sites of atopic eczema

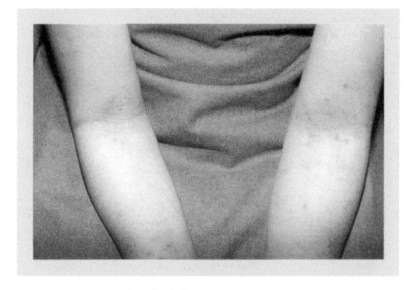

Figure 38 Involvement of the ante-cubital fossae, another classical site

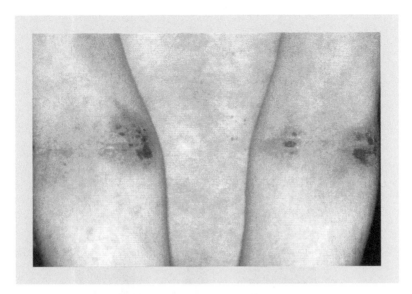

Figure 39 Involvement of the ante-cubital fossae with excoriations, a feature of atopic eczema

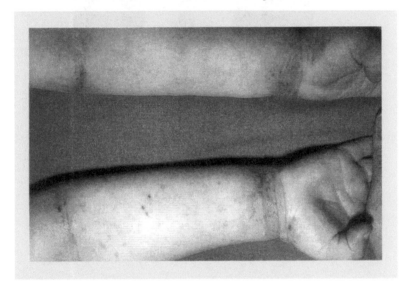

Figure 40 Symmetrical involvement of the wrists and antecubital fossae in atopic eczema

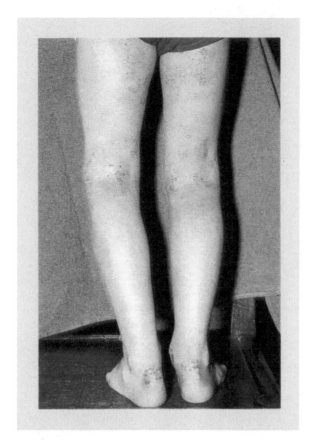

Figure 41 Symmetrical involvement of the ankles, popliteal fossae and thighs

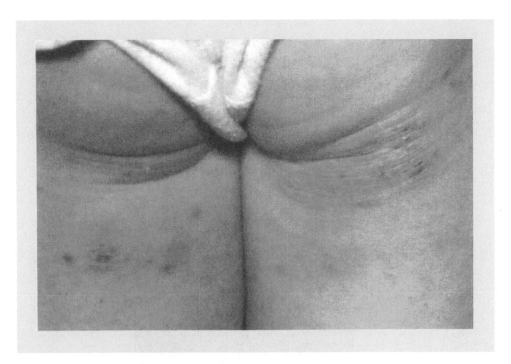

Figure 42 Involvement of the gluteal folds, a common site in atopic eczema

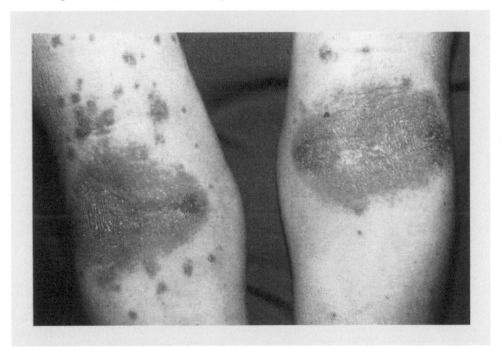

Figure 43 Acute atopic eczema in the central cubital fossae with satellite lesions developing

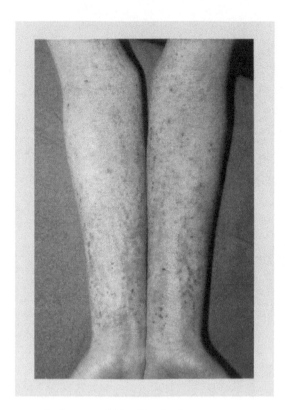

Figure 44 Extensive confluent atopic eczema on the forearms. Lichenification is present

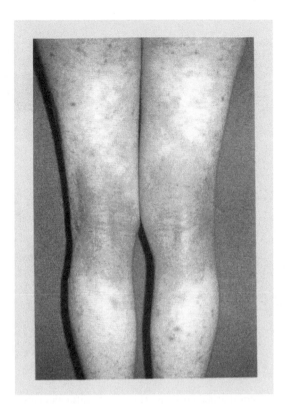

Figure 45 Extensive and excoriated eczema on the back of the legs

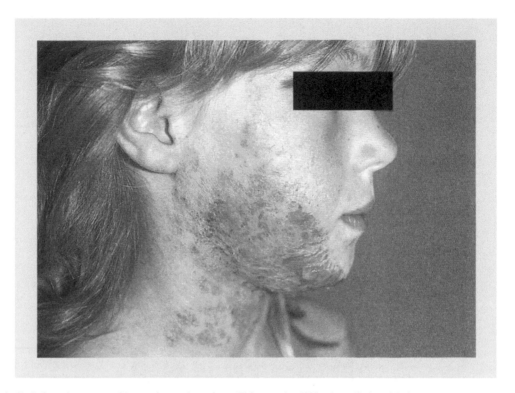

Figure 46 Secondarily infected eczema with crusting and erosions. This may be difficult to distinguish from acute eczema

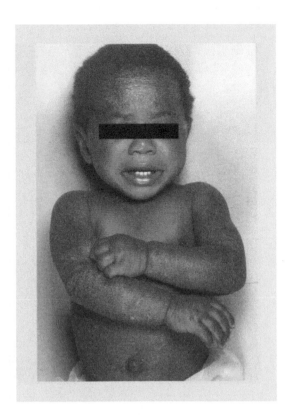

Figure 47 Lichenified patches of atopic eczema in a black child

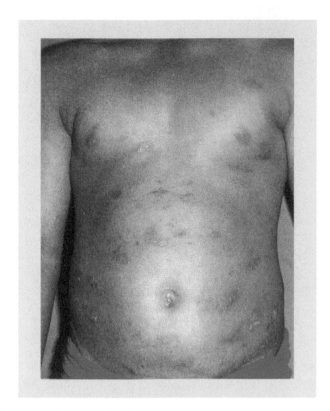

Figure 48 Lichenified eczema. Lichenification is common in black children

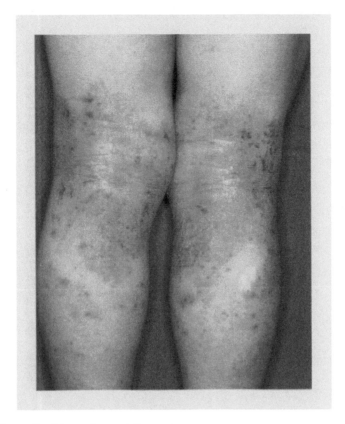

Figure 49 Lichenified eczema in the popliteal fossae in an adult

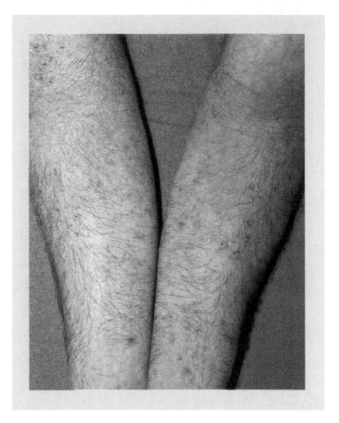

Figure 50 Extensive red, scaly and excoriated lichenified eczema in the antecubital fossae and flexor forearms

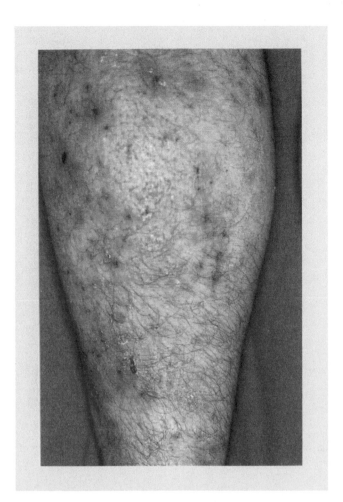

Figure 51 The common appearance of excoriated lichenified eczema, as seen in adults

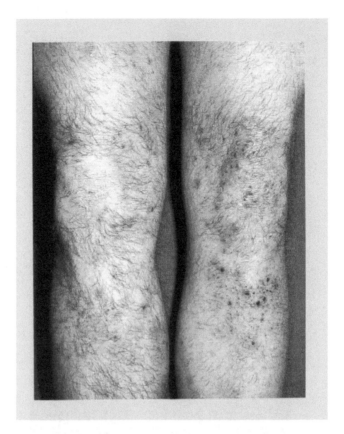

Figure 52 A different pattern and site of excoriated papular atopic eczema on the extensor surfaces of the knees in an adult

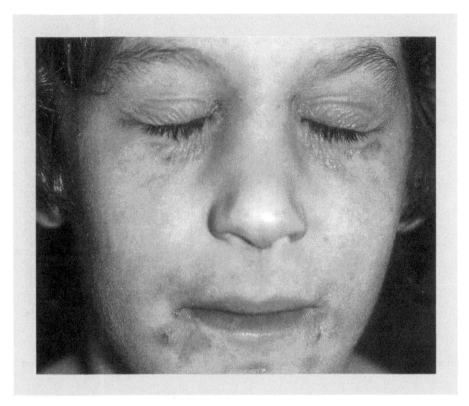

Figure 53 Swelling, redness and scaling of the eyelids and surrounding skin, a common manifestation of atopic eczema in adults

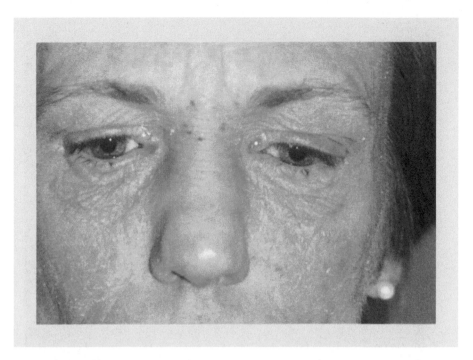

Figure 54 Lichenification with redness and scaling in chronic atopic eczema. The eyelids particularly are involved

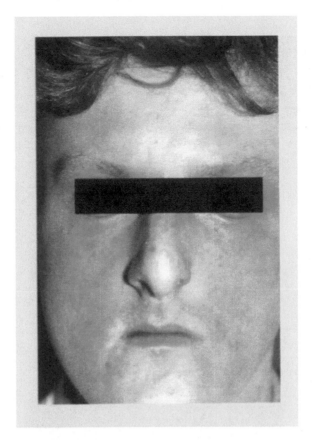

Figure 55 Confluent redness and scaling of the face in adult atopic eczema

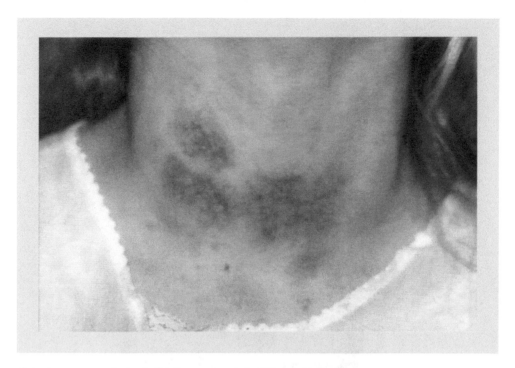

Figure 56 Patches of atopic eczema on the neck. Crusts are present, denoting acute disease

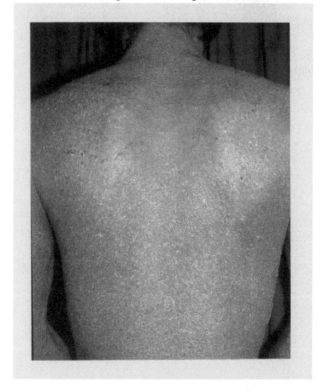

Figure 57 Confluent eczema on the neck and face and patches on the chest

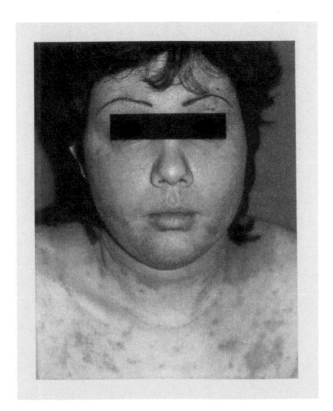

Figure 58 Erythrodermia. The entire skin surface is affected by eczema, a rare manifestation of atopic eczema

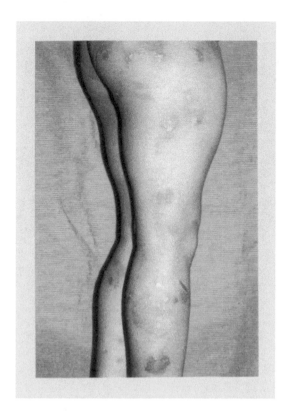

Figure 59 Hyperpigmentation in lichenified plaques. This feature is more common in Asians and black people

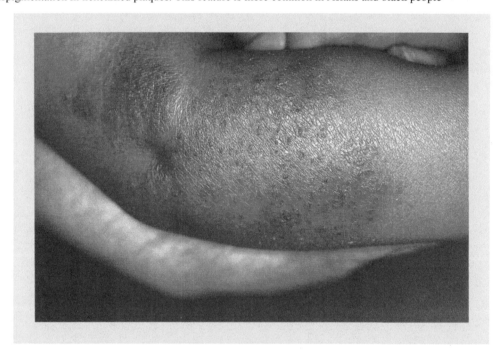

Figure 60 Hyperpigmentation in association with atopic eczema in an infant

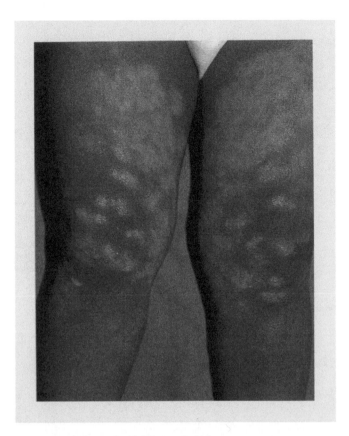

Figure 61 Hypopigmentation at sites of previous eczema which have cleared

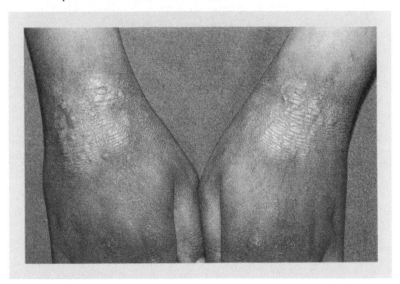

Figure 62 Lichenified patches of eczema associated with loss of pigment. Note that the surrounding skin with less severe eczema shows increased pigmentation

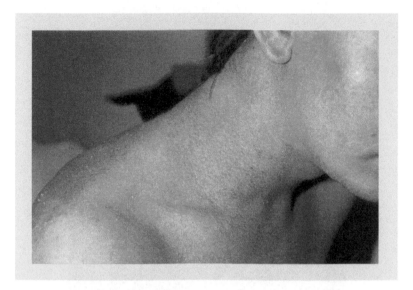

Figure 63 Reticulate pigmentation on the neck in chronic adult eczema

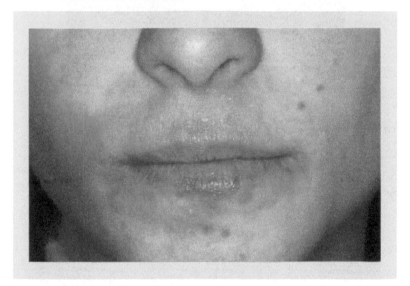

Figure 64 Dry, red, scaling lips with surrounding perioral eczema

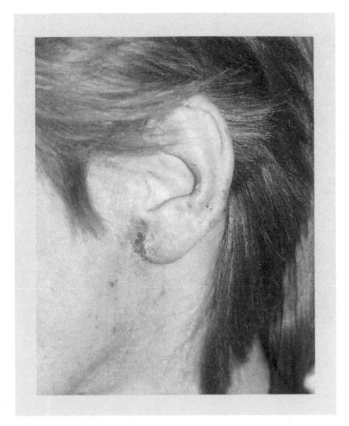

Figure 65 Fissuring, redness and scaling at the base of the pinna, a common site in atopic eczema

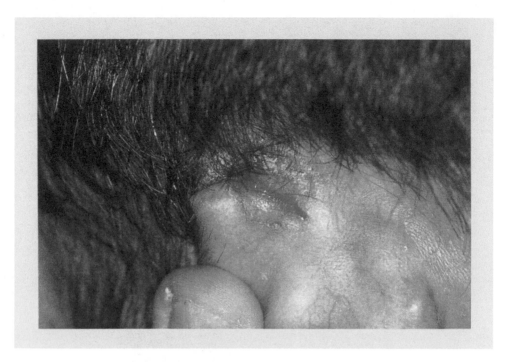

Figure 66 Red scaling and fissuring in the cleft behind the pinna

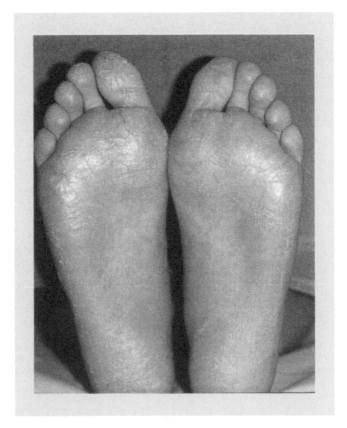

Figure 67 'Shiny foot' syndrome or juvenile plantar dermatosis. Involvement is mainly on the ball of the foot and plantar surfaces of the toes

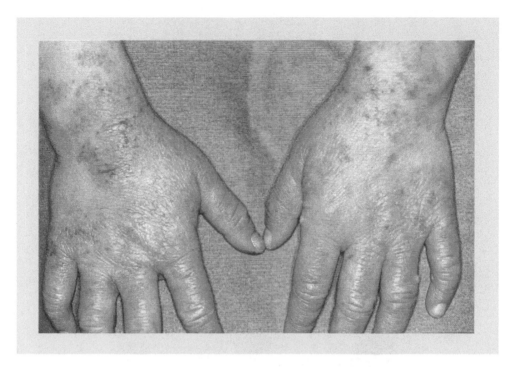

Figure 68 Redness, scaling and fissuring on the back of the hands in atopic eczema. Viral warts are present at the base of the left second finger and on the left fourth finger

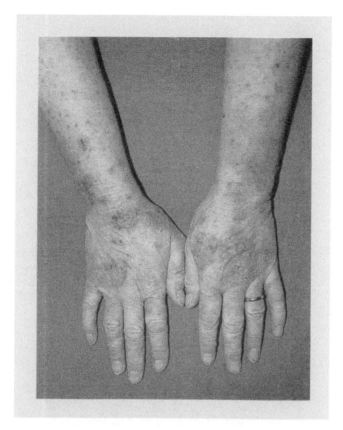

Figure 69 Lichenified excoriated patches of eczema on the back of the hands in an adult

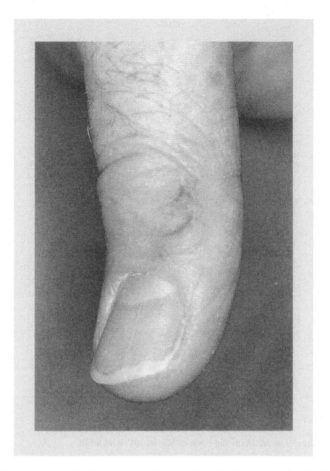

Figure 70 Fissuring in a patch of atopic eczema. This is a common feature when the fingers are involved

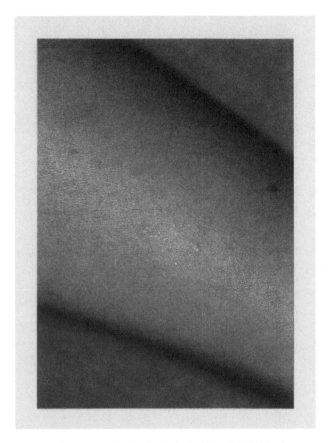

Figure 71 Pityriasis alba: this is most commonly seen on the cheeks in dark-skinned individuals

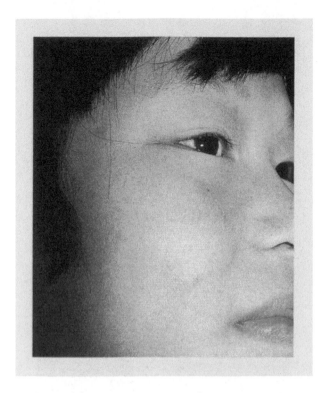

Figure 72 Discoid papular eczema

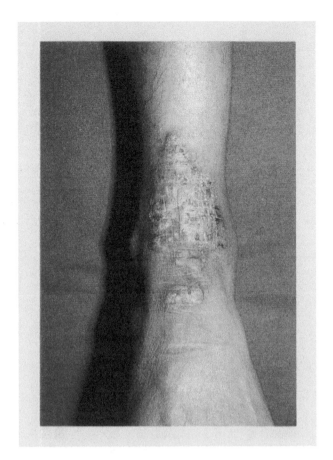

Figure 73 Lichen simplex: localized patch of chronic eczema associated with persistent excoriation

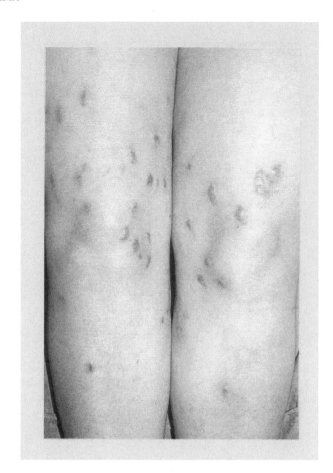

Figure 74 Prurigo nodularis: excoriated nodular lesions

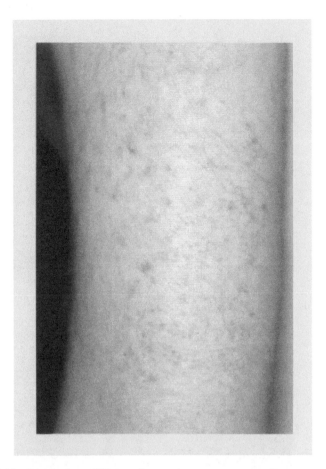

Figure 75 Keratosis pilaris: scaly follicular papules, which are often erythematous

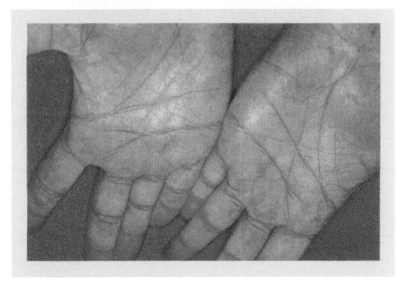

Figure 76 Increased linearity of the palms in atopic eczema

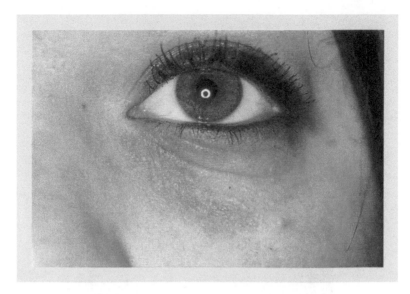

Figure 77 Dennie-Morgan fold under the eye in atopic eczema

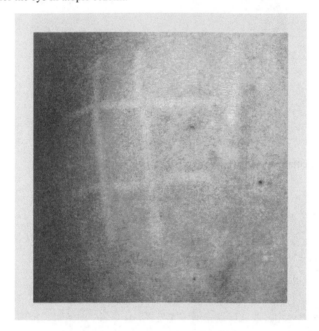

Figure 78 White dermographism: white lines are produced from pressure, with a blunt instrument, in an eczematous area

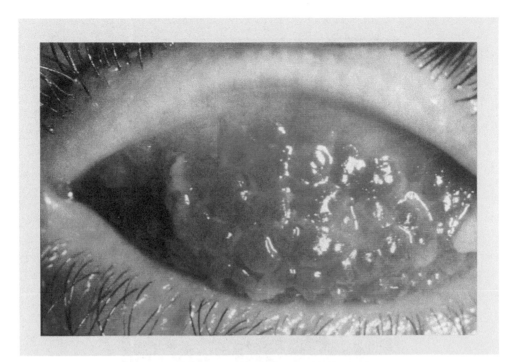

Figure 79 Severe allergic conjunctivitis. Eversion of upper eyelid

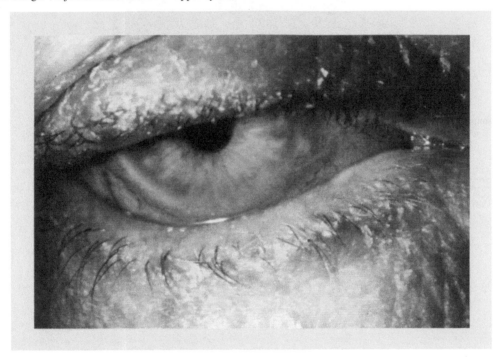

Figure 80 Keratoconjunctivitis: lichenified scaly/crusted eyelids

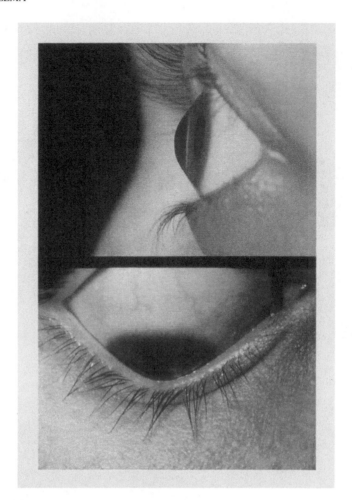

Figure 81 Keratoconus: bulging of the cornea

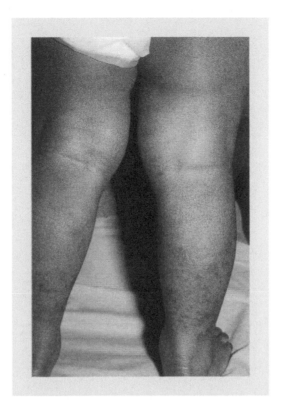

Figure 82 Dry scaly skin in ichthyosis vulgaris. Sparing of the flexures is a characteristic feature

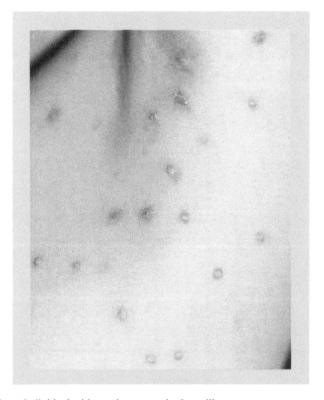

Figure 83 Molluscum contagiosum in an individual with atopic eczema in the axilla

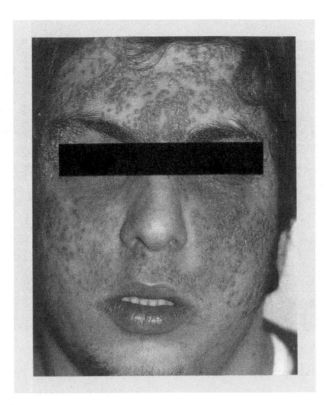

Figure 84 Vesicular eruption of the face in eczema herpeticum

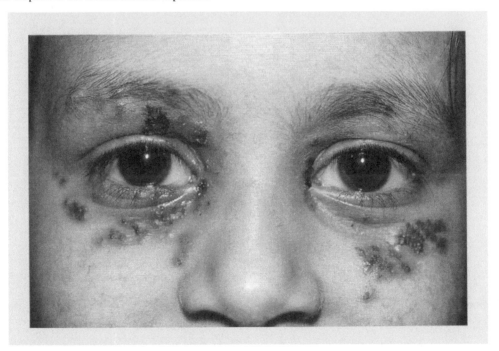

Figure 85 Crusted/vesicular eruption around the eyes in eczema herpeticum

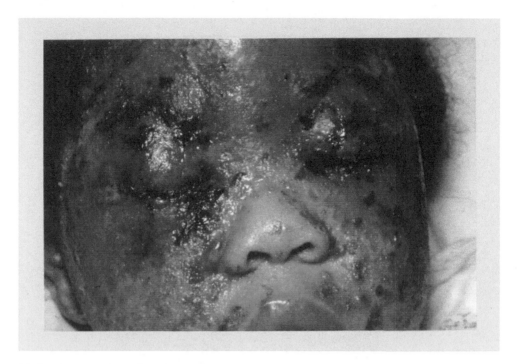

Figure 86 Ulcerated lesions in eczema herpeticum

8
Differential diagnosis

OTHER ECZEMATOUS CONDITIONS

Eczema is divided into endogenous and exogenous types. In the latter, identifiable external substances (allergens and irritants) induce the eczema at the site of contact of the substance. In endogenous eczema, the disease is essentially due to constitutional factors but the exact pathogenetic mechanisms have yet to be elucidated. The classification of endogenous eczema is based on the clinical patterns of the disease. Apart from atopic eczema, the other patterns of endogenous eczemas are seborrheic (infantile and adult forms), discoid or nummular, hand and foot (pompholyx), hypostatic and asteatotic. These clinical patterns are not always distinct, and often there may be combined features of two or even three patterns. In addition, an individual with one pattern of endogenous eczema is more likely to develop another at a different time or in combination.

Seborrheic eczema of infancy

This begins at a younger age than atopic eczema. Seborrheic eczema usually presents between the 2nd and 8th week of life and certainly before 6 months. It may present as cradle cap, with yellowish greasy scales on the scalp, and then spreads to the face and presents as red scaly patches. An alternative presentation is in the napkin area, so-called nappy rash (Figure 87). The eruption may be confined to these areas or spread to involve the neck, axillae (Figure 88) and flexures of the limbs. It presents as confluent red areas. It may also occur on the trunk as red scaly papules, with the scaling having a psoriatic appearance.

Seborrheic eczema of infancy has a good prognosis and, in the majority of infants, the disease will resolve after a few weeks and virtually in all by the age of 1 year. There is no doubt that, in some infants, the pattern of eczema changes from the seborrheic variety into an atopic pattern and, in these instances, the prognosis and course of the eczema are those of an atopic individual.

Discoid eczema

As the name implies, this type of eczema manifests in circular plaques. It most commonly affects the limbs (Figure 89) and the age prevalence is that of young adults. Discoid eczema has a relatively good prognosis, clearing after 2–3 years. In some children with atopic eczema in the flexures, discoid lesions of eczema also occur on the extensor limbs. In these individuals, the question arises as to whether the individuals have both atopic and discoid eczema or whether the lesions are a manifestation of one disease, i.e. atopic eczema. When atopic eczema first presents in infants, it is not uncommon for the lesions first to affect the extensor limbs.

Asteatotic eczema

Asteatotic means without grease. Asteatotic eczema is usually seen in the elderly as the aging process leads to a thinning of the stratum corneum and loss of adhesion between the corneocytes. Keratin is composed of fats and proteins and the loss of fat from the stratum corneum has led to the name asteatotic. Clinically, the defect of the stratum presents as dry scaly skin. Whether the biological defect in the aging skin is the same as in atopic individuals is questionable. It is possible that those elderly persons who develop dry skin are basically atopics.

Asteatotic eczema is most common on the legs (Figure 90), although it may occur on the trunk and arms. The inflammatory component is often linear and the eczema may look like a crazy pavement. It has been given the name eczema craquelé, as the eczema occurs where the skin appears to have cracked.

As with atopic eczema, the asteatotic pattern is more common in cold weather, which exacerbates the tendency of the keratin to crack.

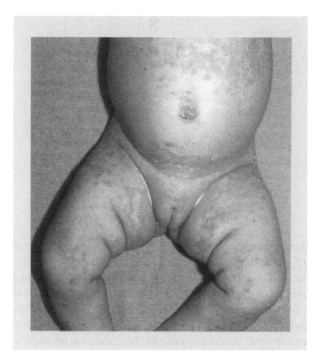

Figure 87 Seborrheic eczema of infancy: well-demar-cated red plaques in the napkin area. Red scaly patches on the trunk and legs are also present

Contact eczema

As has been stated above, contact eczema may be due to chemicals that directly damage the stratum corneum (primary irritants) or due to substances which elicit a true allergic reaction with antigen-specific T-lymphocytes. Primary irritant eczema is most commonly seen on the hands due to overuse of detergents, either from washing-up liquids and household cleaning fluids or occupational use, e.g. in hair-dressing from frequent shampooing without gloves. This type of eczema may be distinguished from atopic hand eczema. The irritant eczema most commonly starts in the web spaces at the base of the fingers and then spreads to involve the fingers and dorsum of the hand (Figure 91). Atopic eczema is common on the back of the fingers and dorsum of the hand but it tends to be more patchy and does not usually involve web spaces. It should be remembered that, because of the inherent defect of the stratum corneum in atopics, irritant eczema tends to be more common in these individuals.

Atopic individuals do not have a higher incidence of allergic contact eczema. In adults, atopic eczema may affect the skin around the eyes and mouth and those individuals often have dry lips. Allergic contact eczema on the face commonly first presents around the eyes (Figure 92), because of the very thin skin at these sites, and is most commonly due to cosmetics. Allergic contact eczema on the lips is usually due to lipstick (Figure 93) and lip balms and, clinically, may be indistinguishable from atopic eczema. It is always worthwhile patch-testing those individuals with an atopic background who develop eczema again in later life, particularly if the pattern suggests a possible allergic cause, rather than simply   labelling the eczema of these patients as recurrence of their atopic disease. It should be remembered that allergic contact eczema is potentially curable if the cause is identified, whereas treatment for atopic eczema is purely suppressive.

SYNDROMES WITH ECZEMATOUS ERUPTIONS

Wiskott-Aldrich syndrome

This is a rare X-linked recessive disorder. The gene for the disease has been mapped to the short arm of the X-chromosome. It is characterized by eczema and thrombocytopenic purpura with associated bleeding and recurrent infection. The eczema usually occurs in the first month of life and affects the scalp, face, flexures and napkin area and is often indistinguishable from atopic eczema. The diagnosis of Wiskott-Aldrich syndrome becomes apparent when the other features become manifest.

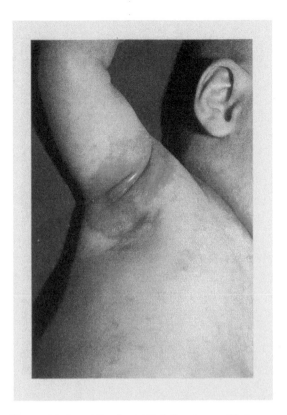

Figure 88 The flexures of the neck and axillae are common sites for seborrheic eczema of infancy

Netherton's syndrome

This is a rare autosomal recessive disorder. It is characterized by a generalized erythroderma soon after birth, much earlier than atopic eczema develops. The atopic features include flexural accentuation and pruritus. There is often a family history of atopy and the individuals may have raised IgE levels.

NON-ECZEMA DISORDERS

Hypertrophic lichen planus

Hypertrophic lichen planus on the legs can resemble lichen simplex lesions of atopic individuals (Figure 94). Both may present as purplish plaques, varying from 1 to 10 cm. The lichen planus lesion may occur anywhere on the lower leg, but lichen simplex is most common on the anterior or lateral aspect just above the ankle.

Psoriasis

Psoriasis is rare in infants and children, which is the most common age group for atopic eczema. When psoriasis does occur in childhood, it often affects the genitalia, groins, and axillae. It is distinguished from eczema by the sharp line of demarcation occurring between the affected and non-affected skin (Figure 95). Psoriasis also tends to be more red, and crusting is not usually a feature.

Guttate psoriasis is usually seen in children and young adults but characteristically affects the trunk, with small red scaly papules, and there is often a history of a streptococcal sore throat 2 weeks before the rash. Guttate psoriasis is not usually confused with atopic eczema. In adults when psoriasis itches and is excoriated, the distinction between psoriatic and eczematous skin lesions may be difficult.

Scabies

The classical lesions of scabies are burrows appearing on the hands and wrists, and papules on the genitalia in males. However, a generalized eruption, which is a reaction to the mite burrowing in the skin, may occur (Figure 96). This

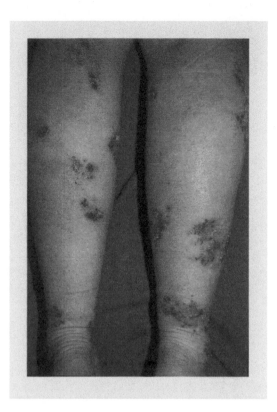

Figure 89 Discoid eczema on the limbs. There are no confluent lichenified patches in the popliteal fossae

generalized eruption has non-specific features of red scaly papules but often shows eczematous features. Thus, patients presenting with eczematous eruptions of recent onset should always be examined for features of scabies.

Acrodermatitis enteropathica

This is a very rare condition, which is thought to be autosomal recessive. It begins 4–6 weeks after weaning, or earlier, if the infant is not breast-fed. The first presentation is a rash around the mouth and on the back of the hands. It is this distribution that often suggests atopic eczema. However, the rash develops blisters and becomes fixed and deep erosions may occur. There is associated hair loss and diarrhea with failure to thrive. The disorder is due to impaired zinc absorption and responds to zinc supplements.

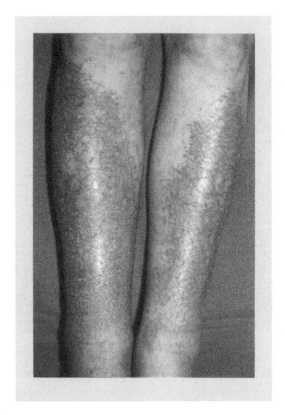

Figure 90 Asteatotic eczema on the legs: superficial cracking of the skin

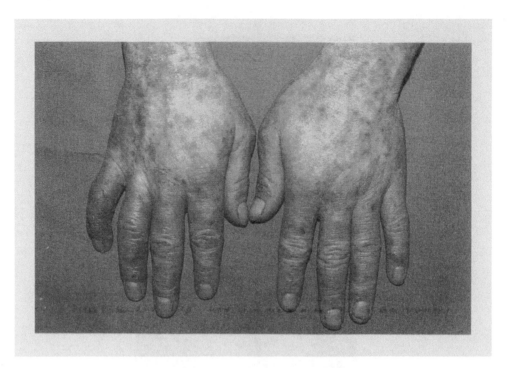

Figure 91 Contact eczema on the back of the hands, involving some of the web spaces and sides of fingers

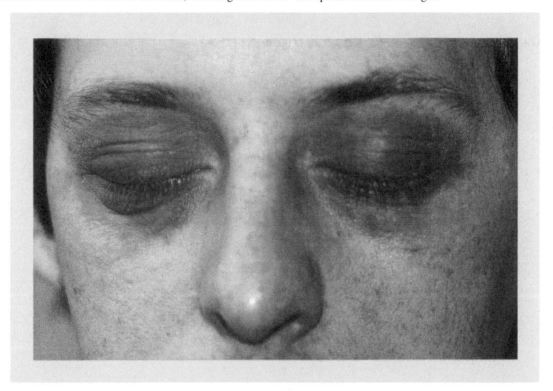

Figure 92 Contact eczema on the eyelids, an allergic reaction to antibiotic eye ointment

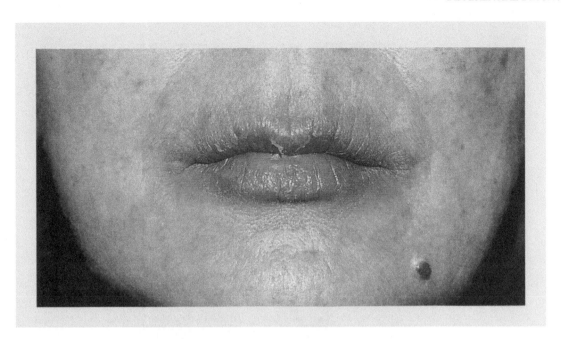

Figure 93 Dry scaly lip due to contact eczema caused by reaction to lipstick

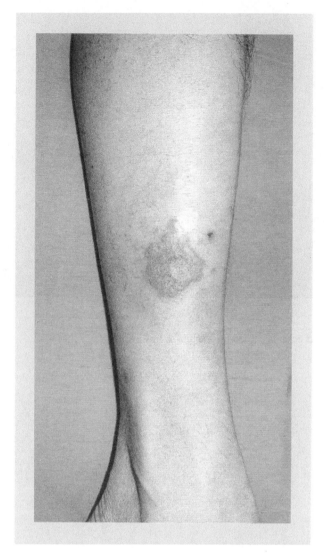

Figure 94 Hypertrophic lichen planus, with similar appearance to lichen simplex (chronic eczema)

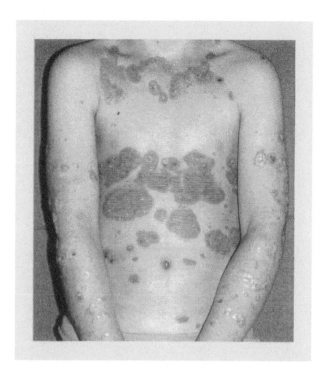

Figure 95 Psoriasis is uncommon in children but may be seen. The well-demarcated plaques are unlike eczema

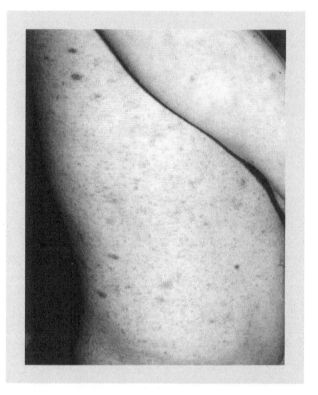

Figure 96 Scabies: generalized scaly erythematous eruption. Large red papules on the trunk may also be seen. They are thought to be the site of the burrowing mite

9
Management

EMOLLIENTS

One of the features of atopic eczema is dry skin associated with an abnormality of the skin barrier or stratum corneum. This dry and abnormal stratum corneum has impaired barrier function and may play a role in the etiology of the eczema by allowing penetration of irritants and microorganisms. Emollients are used to try to create an artificial skin barrier. Essentially, they contain greasy/fatty substances, which form a barrier against penetration of possible irritants and microorganisms. They will also decrease transepidermal water loss and therefore increase hydration of the epidermis.

Emollients have no anti-inflammatory action and thus will have no significant effect on inflamed eczematous skin. They will, therefore, have little effect on irritation. Many so-called emollients are oil-in-water emulsions. The greater the water content, the less greasy they appear. Emollients with high water content have a cooling effect, due to the latent heat of evaporation of the water. The cooling effect may be anti-pruritic, but the lower temperature of the skin will tend to decrease corneocyte bonding and, thus, the barrier function of the stratum corneum, which may be an aggravating factor for eczema. Thus, the main function of emollients is that of possible prevention of eczema rather than a treatment of established disease.

BATHING

Bathing has often been said to aggravate eczema. This may be partly due to the soaps and detergents present in shower gels and bubble baths, which are degreasing agents and which further damage the stratum corneum. In addition, too hot a bath increases the skin temperature, which in turn will increase the blood supply to the skin, leading to further release of inflammatory mediators and increased itching. The latter, in turn, will lead to scratching and aggravation of the eczema. However, bathing may reduce the amount of micro-organisms on the surface of the skin that may play a role in the etiology of eczema.

Emollients containing fatty substances can be added to the bath water to lessen the effect of soaps and detergents on the stratum corneum. A number of substances, which are not soaps or detergents, can be used as soap substitutes. Although they do not possess the cleaning properties of soaps and detergents, they will cause less damage to the stratum corneum, which is already abnormal in atopic eczema. Emulsifying ointment BP is a suitable soap substitute.

CLOTHING

Individuals who are atopic are often intolerant to clothing with 'rough' surfaces next to their skin. Wool and synthetic fibers have rough filaments that induce irritation and make the individual uncomfortable. Articles of clothing made of pure cotton are the most appropriate.

CLIMATE

Cold climates tend to aggravate and warm ones tend to be beneficial for atopic eczema. This is thought to be due in part to the effect of temperature on the corneocyte bonding in the stratum corneum. Corneocyte bonding is temperature-dependent; the lower the temperature, the weaker the bonding. Poor bonding of the skin leads to dryness and impaired barrier function, with aggravation of the eczema.

A warmer climate is also associated with more exposure to sunlight. Ultraviolet light has immuno-suppressive and bacteriocidal properties, both of which are beneficial in decreasing the eczematous process. However, a humid climate, leading to increased sweating and overhydration of the strateum corneum, will aggravate eczema.

DIET

Food allergens have been implicated as a cause of atopic eczema. Parents of children with atopic eczema are often convinced that certain foods are the cause of the disease. However, in the vast majority of patients, elimination diets have not proved helpful. One of the main problems is that there are no reliable tests to predict which foods are responsible for inducing the eczema. In addition, food antigens may illicit a type 1, IgE-mediated reaction in the skin, which is essentially urticarial and associated with irritation but is not an eczematous process.

If parents are convinced that a particular food flares the eczema, then it is reasonable to recommend elimination from the diet for this particular food for a month, followed by gradual re-introduction of the food. If there is definite improvement with an 'elimination' diet and definite deterioration with re-introduction, then it is reasonable to advise elimination of this particular food until the child is older and the eczema is improving. If the elimination diets are pursued, it is important that adequate attention should be paid to dietary supplements, if required.

If dietary antigens are playing a role in the pathogenesis of the eczema, it is unlikely to be one specific antigen. The fault is likely to be in the handling of the antigen in the gut and by the immune system. If there is such a fault, it is likely to apply to several if not all of the dietary antigens, and it is not possible or advisable to try to eliminate them all. Fortunately, the immune system appears to 'mature' with age and the eczema improves and disappears, in the majority, in time.

BREAST-FEEDING

It has been claimed that infants who are breast-fed are less likely to develop atopic eczema. However, there are several reports that infants who are solely breast-fed and have not taken other foods have developed atopic eczema. Therefore, either food is not important in the cause of the eczema or the infant is sensitized to dietary antigens that are present in the mother's milk.

Another benefit of breast-feeding is that secretory IgA is present in breast milk. It has been suggested that secretory IgA binds to dietary antigens and inhibits the absorption of these potential allergens across the immature gut mucosa.

DELAYED INTRODUCTION OF SOLID FOODS

Animal studies have shown that certain antigens, when fed to newborn mice, will invoke humoral and cell-mediated responses, whilst the same allergen given to an adult mouse does not. This observation is also based on an immature response by the gut and immune system to foreign antigens. It has been suggested that the foods most commonly associated with atopic eczema, egg, cow's milk, fish and peanuts, should not be introduced to the diet until the age of 1 year. However, in a study in which fish and citrus fruits were avoided until 1 year, there was no benefit at 3 years follow-up to avoiding allergic reactions to those substances[45].

AVOIDANCE OF FOOD ANTIGENS IN PREGNANCY

It has been suggested that, if the maternal diet in pregnancy was modified so as to reduce the most common food antigens associated with atopic eczema, the measure may prove protective. This environmental manipulation has been tried in pregnancy with measures to avoid the house dust mite antigen and subsequent development of respiratory symptoms in atopy, and was shown to be helpful[46]. Dietary manipulation may prove more difficult in pregnancy since dietary deficiency may develop.

PROBIOTICS

Probiotics are cultures of potentially beneficial bacteria of the healthy gut flora. It has been suggested that specific microbes in the commensal gut flora are more important than infections in promoting anti-allergic responses. These microbes have been associated with the following: Th1 type immunity, generation of TGF-, which suppresses Th2 responses, and induction of oral tolerance and IgA production, an essential component of mucosal immune defence.

In a study of mothers who have had at least one first-degree relative (or partner) with atopic disease (eczema, rhinitis, or asthma), the mother was given lactobacillus GG prenatally and their infants were given it postnatally for 6 months. At the age of 2 years in those receiving lactobacillus GG, the incidence of atopic eczema was 23% vs. 46% in controls[47], a highly significant result. It has recently been shown that this benefit is maintained at 4 years follow-up[48]. The use of probiotics, a simple and safe procedure, certainly looks promising.

AEROALLERGENS

The aeroallergens that have been implicated in atopic eczema are house dust mites, weeds, animal danders, and molds. It has been suggested that these allergens may not only induce eczema by contact with the skin but also through inhalation[49]. However, it should be recalled that the induction of a positive patch test to house dust mite could only be achieved after Sello-tape stripping of the skin, with the removal of the stratum corneum barrier. Thus, it is questionable whether house dust mite antigens can initiate eczema through the skin. It is possible that they may induce eczema through damaged and excoriated skin and thus be an additional antigenic factor in maintaining and exacerbating the eczema after it has been initiated by other antigens (e.g. food).

Two studies have shown improvement in atopic eczema with measures to decrease house dust mite exposure[50, 51]. The latter study was controlled and showed significant improvement in the severity of the eczema. Measures to decrease house dust mite antigens are not easy. Bedding, including pillows, mattresses and quilts, should be covered with allergen-impermeable covers. The mattress and floors should be cleaned with high-filtration vacuum cleaners. Carpets should be replaced by wooden or vinyl floors. Soft toys should be washable and washed at least once a week. Bed linen should be 'hot-washed' weekly. Carpets and soft furnishings should be sprayed with a benzyl benzoate preparation weekly.

Although these measures will decrease the exposure to house dust mites, they may not eradicate them totally. Decrease in house dust mites will not cure atopics, who are likely to have multiple allergies, but they may help, and be worth trying in, infants and children with severe disease.

ANIMALS

Cat, dog and horse dander can cause urticaria (type 1 hypersensitive immune reactions) in atopic subjects. They may also induce asthma and rhinitis. Whether they induce eczema is debatable but, because of the type 1 responses, they will cause irritation and scratching, which themselves may aggravate pre-existing eczema.

Avoidance of the animal is the most appropriate measure. If there is any doubt as to whether removal of the animals will help, the most appropriate procedure is for the child to stay with a relative for 2 weeks and see if the eczema improves and then relapses when they return home.

PSYCHOTHERAPEUTIC MEASURES

Children with atopic diseases are often said to be hyperkinetic. They have boundless energy and seem to need little sleep. Adults with atopic eczema have been reported to have a higher incidence of anxiety, depression, hypochondriasis and hysteria. However, whether these psychological disorders are secondary to their chronic skin problem or whether they are primary factors as part of the atopic diathesis is not certain.

In a controlled trial of psychotherapeutic measures in the treatment of eczema in adults (endogenous but only one with atopic disease), it was shown that the eczema improved in the patients who were receiving psychiatric treatment as opposed to the control group. The treatment consisted of psychotherapy, occasional use of anti-depressants, and training in relaxation and hypnosis[52].

Patients should be referred for psychiatric assessment if there is clear-cut evidence of a psychiatric problem or if the patient raises the question whether their eczema could be due to or aggravated by such problems. It should always be remembered that chronic physical disease itself may lead to psychiatric problems. Clearing the disease may sometimes be the best option.

INVESTIGATIONS

Patients and/or their parents often believe that atopic eczema is due to an allergic response to food and they may well be right. They demand tests to identify the offending food. But the tests available, the 'prick' or epicutaneous tests and RAST for IgE antibodies to food, have not been shown to be helpful in the management (see Chapters 5 and 6). Elimination of foods giving positive tests does not improve the eczema in the majority of individuals. Patch tests in atopic eczema have also been shown not to be helpful in the management of the disease.

TOPICAL DRUGS

When prescribing topical preparations, it is important to consider the vehicle for the drug. Topical preparations may be ointments, creams or lotions. Ointments are composed of fatty substances and tend to be greasy but may remain on the surface of the skin for 8–12 h. Thus, there is a reservoir for the drug for this period of time and the drug will diffuse into the skin during this period. To treat the skin disorder on a continuous basis, the ointment will have to be applied two to three times a day. As a general rule, ointments tend to be the most appropriate vehicle for drugs for dry scaly rashes such as chronic atopic eczema. Another advantage of the ointment base is that it acts as an artificial barrier preventing transepidermal water loss. This hydrates the stratum corneum and enhances the absorption of the drug into the skin.

Creams are oil-in-water emulsions and are approximately 70% water and 30% 'fats'. Creams tend to remain on the surface of the skin for shorter periods than ointments, as the water evaporates when the cream is applied to the skin. The advantage of the cream is that, when the water component evaporates, it cools the skin. This tends to decrease the blood supply to the skin and to lessen the release of inflammatory mediators, thus relieving the itch, but this action is short-lived. Because of the evaporation of the water, the vehicle carrying the drug is on the surface of the skin for a shorter period and, therefore, tends not to be as effective as an ointment, unless it is applied more frequently. To achieve a similar drug reservoir and absorption into the skin as that attained by ointments, creams will have to be applied four times a day.

Lotions will evaporate even more quickly than creams and, therefore, the drug will be on the surface of the skin for a relatively short duration. Lotions may be alcohol- or water-based, depending on the solubility of the drug. In practice, lotions are mainly used for disorders of the scalp because creams and ointments are too greasy and unpleasant to use, unless it is for short periods.

As a rule, ointments are the vehicles of choice for delivery of the drug in eczema. The exceptions are acute weeping eruptions and the intertriginous areas. Creams or lotions should be considered, depending on the situation, because the ointment bases are non-miscible with sweat and tissue fluid.

Apart from the base or vehicle for the drug, it is important to prescribe an appropriate quantity of the drug. All too often, insufficient amounts are given for adequate use. If the disease is extensive, it is important to estimate the percentage of skin surface involved. It takes approximately 30 g to cover the total skin surface of an adult. Thus, if 50% of the body surface is involved, 15 g will be required for each application. The body surface for children has to be estimated, but it should be remembered that the surface area to body weight ratio is proportionally greater in children than in adults. This is of relevance when considering the absorption of the drug into the circulation and possible systemic side-effects.

Corticosteroids

Topical corticosteroids were introduced for dermato-logical conditions in the 1950s and revolutionized the management of atopic eczema. Corticosteroids have a strong anti-inflammatory action and this is the reason why they are so effective in eczema. The cellular effects are due to the binding of the glucocorticosteroids (GCS) to the cytosolic GCS receptor in nucleated cells. Since most cells have these receptors, the effects of the GCS are multiple. Once the steroids have bound to the receptor, there is conformational change in the GCS receptor complex; which moves to the nucleus. The GCS complex now binds to segments of DNA cell glucocorticoid-responsive elements. As a result, certain parts of the genome are affected, leading to increased or decreased transcription, with resulting increased or decreased cytokine production. GCS will also bind to NF-kB, which has been shown to be a regulator for many cytokines and cell adhesion molecules. Binding of GCS to NF-kB will switch off cytokine production, particularly of those cytokines concerned with T-cell-mediated inflammation.

Between the 1950s and 1970s, many new synthetic glucocorticosteroids were produced and introduced into dermatology. The aim was to make these steroids more potent and, therefore, better anti-inflammatory agents. However, the more potent the anti-inflammatory effect, the more potent were the effects on collagen and fibroblasts. One of the actions of corticosteroids is to break down collagen and inhibit fibroblasts, which synthesize collagen. The loss of existing collagen and inhibition of new collagen formation have the clinical effect of making the skin thinner, which is the main side-effect of topical steroids.

When using topical corticosteroids, there are three points to be considered. First, and most important, is the strength of the steroids, second, the site(s) to be treated and, third, the age of the patient.

Strength of topical corticosteroids

When using topical glucocorticosteroids, it is imperative that the physician knows the strength of the steroid. Corticosteroid activity is assessed biologically by the vasoconstrictor test and the fibroblast inhibition assay. The range of activity varies enormously and on some assays, if the weakest glucocorticosteroid is graded as 1 unit, then the strongest is 600 times more potent. It was the failure to appreciate this wide variation in steroid activity that led to side-effects becoming so common in the late 1960s and 1970s. Since then, the opinion of the general public is against steroids and they often refuse to use them. Topical steroids have been placed into four groups, depending on their activity, and have been designated as weak, moderate, strong, and very strong[53]. This has enabled physicians to stop the abuse of topical steroids. It is important to remember that, when prescribing topical steroids, side-effects are proportional to the strength of steroid x duration of use.

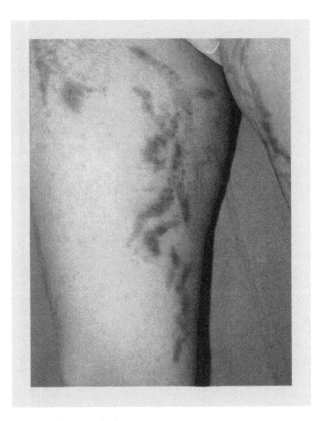

Figure 97 Striae, caused by long-term use of very strong topical steroids

Site

The importance of site is highlighted by the fact that the skin is not of uniform thickness. In areas where the skin is very thin, e.g. face, there will be, first, greater absorption of the steroid and, second, a greater risk of side-effects due to the presence of less collagen in the dermis. Other sites where the skin is relatively thin are the neck and intertriginous areas, and genitalia. As a general rule, the thinner the skin, the weaker the steroid should be.

Another important aspect of site to consider is the differences at the intertriginous areas. Not only is the skin relatively thin but, because the skin surfaces are in contact, the sweat does not evaporate so easily as at other sites and this leads to increased hydration of the stratum corneum, producing greater absorption of the steroid.

Age

It should be stressed that infants have thinner skins than children. The thinner the skin, the more risk of thinning the skin further with steroids. In addition, there is a risk of greater absorption of the steroid and possible systemic side-effects. Thus, very potent steroids should be avoided in infants. It should be remembered that thinning of the skin is part of the aging process. This is important when using topical steroids in patients over the age of 75, who are likely to have thin skins.

How to use topical corticosteroids in eczema

It is important to use the weakest possible steroid to treat the eczema and for the shortest period of time. However, the aim of treatment is to try to clear the eczema and induce a remission. The strength of the steroid will depend on the severity of the eczema and the age of the patient. In infants, weak- or moderate-strength topical steroids are usually effective. Weak ones should be used for the face. They also can be used at other sites as the initial treatment, but the moderate-strength ones may be used for short periods (i.e. up to 2 weeks) if the eczema is severe

In children, if the eczema is severe, the strong topical steroids are acceptable for the trunk and limbs for periods of up to 2 weeks and not more often than every 2 months. Similarly, in adults, very strong topical steroids may be used for a 2-week period but not more frequently than every 2 months. This can be referred to as 'the rule of 2': twice daily for 2 weeks but not more frequently than every 2 months. The aim of using potent or very potent topical steroids for short periods is to try to induce a remission. There is evidence that this does occur.

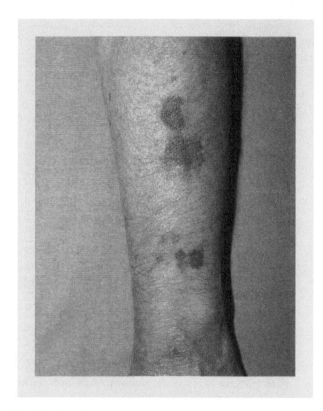

Figure 98 Purpura seen in thinning of the skin due to long-term use of strong topical steroids

Auto-sensitization is seen in eczematous conditions. This phenomenon is the development of eczema at distant sites from the original patch of acute eczema. Appropriate treatment, in which the goal is to clear the eczema, is more effective than trying to 'damp down' the eczema with weak and ineffective topical steroids.

If the eczema clears, then no topical steroids should be used. The patient should be informed that steroids should not be used as a preventative but only as treatment to clear the disease. If the eczema clears in the majority of the areas with strong/ very strong topical steroids after a 2-week period, but there are small areas remaining, then it is permissible to continue for another week or two for these lesions. If and when the eczema recurs, patients should use weak- or moderate-strength topical steroids in the first instance. The more potent ones should be reserved for severe disease.

Side-effects

Local If topical steroids are used correctly, side-effects should not occur. Side-effects are due to the use of too strong a preparation for too long and at the wrong site. Side-effects are due to the thinning of skin resulting from collagen atrophy in the dermis. Clinically, this may present as striae (Figure 97), purpura (Figure 98), spontaneous 'bruising' and telangiectasia (Figure 99). If potent topical steroids are applied to the face, they may give rise to so-called peri-oral eczema, which is exaggerated when the patients attempt to discontinue the steroids. The appearances of the eruption are similar to rosacea, with small red papules and pustules, but the distribution is different.

Systemic absorption If large quantities of potent topical steroids are applied to extensive areas over long periods of time, enough steroid may be absorbed to cause suppression of the pituitary-adrenal axis and even Cushingoid features. In adults, the suppression of the pituitary-adrenal axis would require at least 50 g of clobetasol propionate (a very strong topical steroid) to be used in 1 week. It would probably take some months for Cushingoid features to appear. To produce similar effects with strong topical steroids would require greater quantities (i.e. 300 g per week). These side-effects are unlikely to be seen with moderate or weak topical steroids in adults. However, in children, because of their thinner skin and greater ratio of skin surface to body weight, there is a greater risk of these side-effects.

Avoidance of side-effects The two golden rules for the limitation of side-effects are:

(1) Topical steroids should not be given on repeat prescriptions. Patients must be seen by their doctor if further supplies are required;
(2) Strong/very strong steroids should not be used as maintenance therapy.

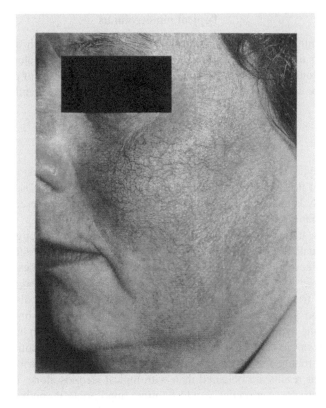

Figure 99 Telangiectasia on the face due to strong topical steroids

Intralesional corticosteroids

These have a limited role in atopic eczema in adults. The indication for intralesional corticosteroids is the presence of resistant patches of lichenified eczema. This treatment should only be carried out by a physician experienced in this technique.

Topical tacrolimus

Tacrolimus (FK 506) is a potent immunosuppressive agent, which has been used in transplantation to prevent organ rejection. It acts by binding to an intracellular binding protein (FK BP) and forming a complex, which inhibits the enzyme calcineurin. This enzyme is necessary for activation pathways requiring a rise in intracellular calcium. Drugs that act in this way are referred to as calcineurin inhibitors. This failure to raise intracellular calcium levels results in a block of the signal transduction required for cytokine gene expression. This leads to inhibition of cytokine production, including IL-2, IL-3, IL-4, IFN- and TNF- . Thus, both Th1 and Th2 cytokine production, an integral part of eczema, is blocked.

Tacrolimus is a smaller molecule than cyclosporin and is absorbed into the skin. It has been shown to be effective in treating atopic eczema[54] and has recently been given a licence for use in atopic eczema in adults and children over 2 years of age for short-term use and intermittent long-term use. Compared to topical steroids, tacrolimus appears to be as effective as a moderate-strength topical steroid. Its place in the management of atopic eczema would appear to be for severe eczema on the face resistant to weak topical steroids. It may also have a role in the treatment of intertriginous areas, where potent topical steroids are best avoided.

Side-effects

In approximately one-quarter of patients, there is a burning sensation after application of the drug. This tends to wear off with continued use.

The more worrying potential side-effects are those associated with immunosuppression. These would include impaired immunity to viral infection, e.g. herpes simplex, and the possible long-term effects on the development of skin cancers, as seen with systemic immunosuppressive agents. It is too early to have any information on these side-effects.

Topical pimecrolimus

This is another calcineurin inhibitor with immuno-suppressive properties similar to those of tacrolimus. Recent treatments have shown it to be effective in treating atopic eczema when compared to vehicle alone[55]. However, when compared to betametha-sone 17-valerate (a strong topical steroid), it was less effective[56]. The place of pimecrolimus in the management of atopic eczema would appear to be similar to that of tacrolimus. The side-effects, real and potential, are the same as those of tacrolimus.

ANTISTAPHYLOCOCCAL TREATMENT

As has been mentioned previously, *S.aureus* is present in over 90% of atopic eczema lesions. However, whether the organism plays a role in the pathogenesis of the diseases or whether it is secondary to the eczema is as yet not decided. After successful treatment with both topical steroids and tacrolimus, the organisms are no longer present[57,58]. These observations seem to imply that the presence of the organism is secondary.

However, in some individuals, the eczema lesions are modified and resemble impetigo, and the picture is referred to as impetiginized eczema. In this situation, there is no doubt that antibiotics, topical and systemic, improve the infected eczema. The appearance reverts to that of eczema. These individuals often have recurrent episodes of impetiginized eczema, implying that they are either *S.aureus* carriers or that they have an inability to deal with these organisms. If there is repeated clinical infection, swabs should be taken from the carrier sites and, if *S.aureus* is present, topical fusidic acid or mupiricin should be applied for at least 6 weeks and swabs taken again to be certain that the organisms have been eradicated. Antiseptic preparations, such as chlorhexidine hydrochloride and benzalkonium chloride added to bath water or to an emollient for use after bathing, will decrease the *S.aureus* content of the skin and may be helpful in preventing recurrent impetiginized eczema.

It is questionable whether the routine use of topical antibiotics combined with topical steroids can be justified. Although there is some evidence that better results are obtained than with topical steroids alone, there is a risk of inducing resistant strains of *S.aureus* with this approach. Antiseptics would be more appropriate if routine antibacterial substances could be shown to definitely improve the eczema.

ANTIVIRAL TREATMENT

One of the more severe complications of atopic eczema is eczema herpeticum (Figures 84–86). This is a widespread eruption due to herpes simplex, which usually begins on the face but may appear on the trunk and limbs. The initial lesions are blisters, which may be umbilicated. When the blisters rupture, they may form erosions, which invariably become secondarily infected with *S.aureus* and become crusted. The diagnosis may be missed and simply thought to be impetiginized eczema. Antiviral treatment with systemic aciclovir or famci-clovir should be given as soon as the diagnosis is suspected. It is important not to delay treatment and wait for confirmation of the infection by laboratory tests. Since secondary infection with *S. aureus* is common, it is advisable to give appropriate systemic antibiotics.

A similar picture to eczema herpeticum may be seen with vaccinia virus. Smallpox has been eradicated and vaccination is no longer required. However, because of the threat of bioterrorism with smallpox virus, vaccination may be reintroduced and physicians should be aware of so-called eczema vaccinatum, following vaccination with vaccinia virus. The treatment is the same as that for eczema herpeticum.

ANTIFUNGAL TREATMENT

The yeast organism *Pityrosporum orbiculare* has been claimed to play a role in atopic eczema, particularly of the head and neck. It has been maintained that appropriate antifungal treatment improves the eczema at these sites[35]. Topical or systemic triazole antifungal preparations are the most appropriate.

ULTRAVIOLET LIGHT

It has been known for many years that natural sunlight is beneficial for atopic eczema. In certain countries, e.g. Northern European ones, which do not have much natural sunlight, artificial sources of ultraviolet light have been developed and have been shown to be helpful for eczema and psoriasis. In eczema, the role of ultraviolet light may be twofold. First, it has immunosuppressive properties that interfere with the function of the Langerhans cells (antigen-presenting) and lymphocytes. Second, ultraviolet light has antibacterial properties and will decrease the number of *S.aureus* organisms on the skin.

In countries where natural sunlight is not available, there are currently three forms of ultra- violet light treatment. The first is with high-intensity UVB lamps, so-called narrowband UVB, with the lamps emitting UVB at 311 nm. The second is with high-intensity UVA-1 (340–400 nm). The third is with PUVA. PUVA stands for psoralens+UVA (long-wave ultraviolet light). Psoralens are photo-sensitizers and increase the effect of the ultraviolet light on the skin. The advantage of narrowband UVB is that no tablets are required, compared to treatment with PUVA. Psoralens may cause gastrointestinal symptoms, particularly nausea, and subjects have to be cautious about going into the sun and artificial sources of UVA for up to 6–8 h after taking the drug. If the gastrointestinal upset is severe, it is possible to use psoralens topically. The psoralens are added to bath water and patients lie in the bath for 10 min prior to receiving their UVA treatment.

Narrowband UVB and PUVA should be reserved for chronic and persisting eczema that is not responsive to topical measures. It is not really suitable for infants and young children. There is some evidence (as with very potent topical steroids) that ultraviolet light regimes may induce remissions[59].

Climate therapy

Treatment of skin disease at the Dead Sea Center has a beneficial effect on both psoriasis and eczema. The Dead Sea Center has two unique properties. First, it is 400 m below sea level and is surrounded by mountains. The water vapor from the evaporation of the sea is retained in the area and the water droplets filter out the UVB rays and not the UVA. The UVB rays (middle-wave length) are the rays that induce the sunburn response. The UVA rays, which are not filtered out, do not cause sunburn but have a beneficial effect on eczema and psoriasis and the patients can stay on the beach all day.

The second advantageous effect of the Dead Sea is the high concentration of salt and other minerals that increase the hydration of the streateum corneum. However, any cracks or fissures from the eczema will cause stinging when the concentrated salt water is in contact with the skin.

SYSTEMIC TREATMENT

This is reserved for severe eczema not responsive to topical measures and ultraviolet light. Fortunately, the number of patients with atopic eczema not controlled by these measures is very few. The drugs used are systemic corticosteroids and immuno-suppressive ones.

Corticosteroids

These are highly effective and will suppress the eczema. However, if the eczema is severe, it tends to relapse when the steroids are discontinued. Because of the long-term side-effects of systemic steroids, they are not advocated for long-term treatment. Systemic steroids are indicated in short courses for treatment of a flare-up of atopic eczema. Their advantage is that they act quickly and, for short courses, are relatively safe.

Usually prednisolone, 30 mg daily, is sufficient to suppress the eczema and treatment should be tailed off after 2 weeks.

Cyclosporin

This is a potent immunosuppressive drug that was used to stop rejection of transplanted organs. Its primary site of action is on activated T-lymphocytes, where it will block cytokine production. It is effec-tive in atopic eczema with an initial dose of 3 mg/kg/day. Cyclosporin has three main side-effects. First, it is nephrotoxic. In periods of up to 2 years, the nephrotoxicity appears to be reversible but, if continued for longer periods, the risk of permanent impairment of renal function increases with the duration of use. Second, cyclosporin may induce hypertension. Thus, a patient's renal function and blood pressure must be monitored on a regular basis. The third complication is that long-term immunosuppression may lead to the development of malignancy particularly of the skin in sun-exposed areas.

Azathioprine

This is an immunosuppressive agent, whose mode of action is the inhibition of DNA synthesis and which thus inhibits mitosis. Azathioprine reduces both T-and B-cell proliferation. Its main side-effect is bone marrow suppression. Patients who have low levels of the enzyme thiopurinemethyl transferase are particularly at risk. This enzyme should be measured before starting treatment with azathioprine. If the drug is taken long-term, there is a risk of malig-nancies, particularly lymphomas and skin cancers.

Azathioprine has been shown to have beneficial effects in atopic eczema but there have been no controlled trials and it is not as effective as cyclosporin. The therapeutic effect of immuno-suppressive drugs in eczema is proportional to their efficiency as immunosuppressive agents.

Mycophenolate mofetil

This is another immunosuppressive drug, whose mode of action is via inhibition of purine bio-synthesis. It has been shown to be effective in atopic eczema[60]. As with all current immunosuppressive agents, there are serious potential side-effects, which include bone marrow suppression and the risks of malignancy with long-term immunosuppression.

BIOLOGICAL AGENTS

Monoclonal antibodies

In an attempt to circumvent the side-effects of immunosuppressive drugs, a number of monoclonal antibodies have been produced directed against the cytokines and cytokine receptors involved in immune responses in chronic inflammatory diseases, e.g. rheumatoid arthritis, Crohn's disease, and psoriasis. The monoclonal antibodies that have been used are against TNF- , TNF- receptor, and IL-2 receptor. The results so far are promising. The treatment is not without side-effects and the long-term hazards are not known, but, if the patients are immunosuppressed, the risk of malignancy exists, as with immunosuppressive drugs. As yet, there are no reports of these monoclonal antibodies in the treatment of eczema but they are likely to be effective.

Cytokines

Recombinant IFN- , which down-regulates Th2 responses, has been reported to be of benefit in atopic eczema[61]. However, IFN- is a constituent cytokine in the chronic phase of atopic eczema and, in this instance, recombinant IFN- may aggravate the eczema.

IL-10 is an inhibitory cytokine in inflammation mediated by both Th1 and Th2 cytokines. 11–10 has been reported to improve psoriasis and it is likely to have a similar effect in atopic eczema. Interestingly, in schistosomiasis infection (a parasitic infection) which invokes Th2 responses, the incidence of atopic eczema is very low, and it has been suggested that this may be due to the fact that the infestation also invokes IL-10 production[62].

Monoclonal antibody to IgE

Recently, it has been shown that a monoclonal antibody to IgE can block IgE binding to receptors on mast cells and basophils. This observation has led to a study in which peanut-sensitive individuals were given the monoclonal antibody to IgE and then challenged with increasing amounts of peanut antigen[63]. It was found that the antibody raised the amount of antigen required to initiate a type 1 hypersensitivity response. In atopic eczema, it is thought that the IgE bound to antigen-presenting cells may be involved in the pathogenesis of the eczema. In theory, it may be possible to develop an antibody to that part of the IgE molecule that binds to a receptor on the antigen-presenting cell, and thus inhibit the development of eczema.

THE FUTURE

Atopic eczema may well be an antigen-driven disorder but the primary fault is likely to be in the immune response to multiple foreign proteins, e.g. food and aeroallergens. The disease is unlikely to be due to a single allergen. The fact that the majority of patients with atopic eczema 'grow out' of their disorder implies a different response by the immune system as the individual matures. Efforts to block or alter this abnormal response to foreign antigens are required. The initial observation on the use of probiotics looks promising and appears to carry little risk. Induction of tolerance by other methods long sought by clinical immunologists may well be developed as our knowledge on immune mechanisms increases.

References

1. Coco AF, Cooke RA. On the classification of the phenomenon of hypersensitivities. *J Immunol* 1923; 8:163–82
2. Bos JD. Atopiform dermatitis. *Br J Dermatol* 2002; 147:426–9
3. Hanifin JM, Rajka G. Diagnostic features of atopic dermatitis. *Acta Derm Venereol Suppl (Stockh)* 1980; 92:44–7
4. Williams HC, Burney PGJ, Pembroke AC, *et al.* The UK working party diagnostic criteria for atopic dermatitis. III. Independent hospital validation. *Br J Dermatol* 1994; 131:406–16
5. McNally N, Phillips D. Geographical studies of atopic dermatitis. In Williams HC, ed. *Atopic Dermatitis.* Cambridge: Cambridge University Press, 2000:71–84
6. Williams HC, Robertson CE, Stewart AW, *et al.* Worldwide variations in the prevalence of symptoms of atopic eczema in the international study of asthma and allergies in childhood. *J Allergy Clin Immunol* 1999; 103:125–38
7. Charman C, Williams HC. Epidemiology. In Bieber T, Leung DYM, eds. *Atopic Dermatitis.* New York: Marcel Dekker, 2002:21–42
8. Herd RM. The morbidity and cost of atopic dermatitis. In Williams HC, ed. *Atopic Dermatitis.* Cambridge: Cambridge University Press, 2000:85–95
9. Schultz-Larsen F, Hanifin JM. Secular change in the occurrence of atopic dermatitis. *Acta Derm Venereol Suppl (Stockh)* 1992; 176: 7–12
10. Schultz-Larsen F. Atopic dermatitis, a genetic-epidemiological study in a population-based twin sample. *J Am Acad Dermatol* 1993; 28:719–23
11. Kay J, Gawkrodger DJ, Mortimer MJ, *et al.* The prevalence of childhood atopic eczema in a general population. *J Am Acad Dermatol* 1994; 30:35–9
12. Williams HC, Strachan DP. The natural history of childhood eczema: observations from the 1958 British Cohort Study. *Br J Dermatol* 1998; 120:834–9
13. Vickers CFH. The natural history of atopic eczema. *Acta Derm Venereol Suppl (Stockh)* 1980; 92:113–15
14. Williams HC, Wuthrich B. The natural history of atopic dermatitis. In Williams HC, ed. *Atopic Dermatitis.* Cambridge: Cambridge University Press, 2000:43–59
15. Rystedt L. Long-term follow-up in atopic dermatitis. *Acta Derm Venereol Suppl (Stockh)* 1986; 114:117–20
16. Larsen FS. Genetic epidemiology of atopic eczema. In Williams HC, ed. *Atopic Dermatitis.* Cambridge: Cambridge University Press, 2000:113–24
17. Cookson WO, Moffat MF. The genetics of atopic dermatitis. *Curr Opin Allergy Clin Immunol* 2002; 5:383–7
18. Cookson WO, Ubhi B, Lawrence R, *et al.* Genetic linkage of childhood atopic dermatitis to psoriasis susceptibility loci. *Nature Genet* 2001; 27:372–9
19. Cox HE, Moffat MF, Faux JA, *et al.* Association of atopic dermatitis to the beta subunit of the high affinity immunoglobulins E receptor. *Br J Dermatol* 1998; 138:182–7
20. Schultz-Larsen F. Genetic epidemiology of atopic dermatitis. In Williams HC, ed. *Atopic Dermatitis.* Cambridge: Cambridge University Press, 2000:113–24
21. Cookson WO. The alliance of genes and environment in asthma and allergy. *Nature* 1999; 402:B5–11
22. Prausnitz C, Kustner H. Studien die uber die Ueberemptindlichkeit. *Zentralbl Bakteriol* 1921;86:160–9
23. Werfel T, Kapp A. T cells in atopic dermatitis. In Bieber T, Leung DYM, eds. *Atopic Dermatitis.* New York: Marcel Dekker, 2002: 241–66
24. Scalabrin DMF, Baubek S, Perzanowski MS, *et al.* Use of specific IgE in assessing the relevance of fungal and dust mite allergens in atopic dermatitis. A comparison with asthmatic and non-asthmatic control subjects. *J Allergy Clin Immunol* 1999; 104:1273–9
25. Walley AJ, Chavanas S, Moffat MF, *et al.* Gene polymorphism in Netherton and common atopic disease. *Nature Genetics* 2001; 29: 175–8
26. von Bubnoff D, Novak N, Kraft S, *et al.* The central role of FceRI in allergy. *Clin Exp Dermatol* 2003; 28:184–7
27. Zhang Y, Leaves NI, Anderson GG, *et al.* Positional cloning of a quantitative trait locus on chromosome 13q14 that influences immunoglobulin E levels and asthma. *Nature Genet* 2003; 34:181–6
28. Elliott K, Forrest S. Genetics of atopic dermatitis. In Bieber T, Leung DYM, eds. *Atopic Dermatitis.* New York: Marcel Dekker 2002: 81–110
29. David TJ, Patel L, Ewing CI, Stanton RHJ. Dietary factors in established atopic dermatitis. In Williams HC, ed. *Atopic Dermatitis.* Cambridge: Cambridge University Press, 2000:193–201
30. Munkvad M, Danielsen L, Hoj L, *et al.* Antigen-free diet in adult patients with atopic dermatitis. *Acta Derm Venereol (Stockh)* 1984; 64:524–8
31. Devlin J, David TJ, Stanton RHJ. Elemental diet for refractory atopic eczema. *Arch Dis Childh* 1991; 66:93–9
32. Hattevig, G, Kjellman B, Johansson SGO, *et al.* Clinical symptoms and IgE responses to common food problems in atopic and healthy children. *Clin Allergy* 1984; 14:551–9
33. Kleinman RE, Walker WA. Antigen processing and uptake from the intestinal tract. *Clin Rev Allergy* 1984; 2:25–37

34. Sampson HA. Late phase response to food in atopic dermatitis. *Hosp Pract* 1987; 22:111–28

35. Leung DYM, Bieber T. Atopic dermatitis. *Lancet* 2003; 361:151–60

36. Bygum A, Mortz CG, Andersen KE. Atopy patch tests in young adult patients with atopic dermatitis and controls: dose-response relationship, objective reading, reproducibility and clinical interpretation. *Acta Derm Venereol (Stockh)* 2003; 83:18–23

37. Abeck D, Ruzicka T. Bacteria and atopic eczema: merely association or etiologic factor. In Ruzick T, Bing, Przybilla B, eds. *Handbook of Atopic Eczema.* Berlin: Springer-Verlag, 1991:212–20

38. Motala C, Potter PC, Weinberg EG, *et al.* Anti *Staphylococcus aureus*-specific IgE in atopic dermati-tis. *J Allergy Clin Immunol* 1986; 78:583–9

39. Skov L, Olsen JV, Giorno R, *et al* Application of staphylococcal enterotoxin B on normal and atopic skin induces upregulation of T cells by a super antigen mediated mechanism. *J Allergy Clin Immunol* 2000;105:820–6

40. Ong PY, Ohtake T, Brandt T, *et al.* Endogenous antimicrobial peptides and skin infections in atopic dermatitis. *N Engl J Med* 2002; 347:1151–60

41. Schafer T, Ring J. The possible role of environmental pollution in the development of atopic dermatitis. In Williams HC, ed. *Atopic Dermatitis.* Cambridge: Cambridge University Press, 2000:155–68

42. Alm JS, Swartz J, Lilja G, *et al.* Atopy in children of families with an anthroposophic lifestyle. *Lancet* 1999; 353:1485–8

43. Schultz-Larsen F, Diepgen T, Svensson A. Clinical criteria in diagnosing AD. The Lillehammer Criteria 1994. *Acta Derm Venereol Suppl (Stockh)* 1996; 76:115–19

44. Rajka G. *Atopic Dermatitis.* Philadelphia: Saunders 1975:4–35

45. Saarinen UM, Kajosaari M. Does dietary elimination in infancy prevent or only postpone a food allergy? A study of fish and citrus allergy in 375 children. *Lancet* 1980; 1:166–7

46. Cutovic A, Simpson BM, Simpson A, *et al.* Effect of environmental manipulation in pregnancy and early life on respiratory symptoms and atopy during the first year of life: a randomised trial. *Lancet* 2001; 358:188–93

47. Kalliomaki M, Salminen S, Arvilommi H, *et al.* Probiotics in primary prevention of atopic disease: a random placebo controlled trial. *Lancet* 2001; 357:1076–9

48. Kalliomaki M, Salminen S, Poussa T, *et al.* Probiotics and prevention of atopic disease: 4-year follow-up of a randomised placebo-controlled trial. *Lancet* 2003; 361:1869–71

49. Tupker RA, De Monchy JG, Coenraads PJ, *et al.* Induction of atopic dermatitis by the inhalation of house dust mites. *J Allergy Clin Immunol* 1996; 97:1064–70

50. Roberts DL. House dust mite avoidance and atopicdermatitis. *Br J Dermatol* 1994; 110:735–6

51. Tan BB, Weald DD, Strickland I, *et al.* Double blind controlled trial of effect of house dust mite allergen avoidance on atopic dermatitis. *Lancet* 1996; 347:15–18

52. Brown BG, Bettley FR. Psychiatric treatment of eczema: a controlled trial. *Br Med J* 1971; 2:729–6

53. Fry L. *Dermatology: An Illustrated Guide.* London: Update Publications, 1978:162

54. Paller A, Eichenfield LF, Leung DY, *et al.* A 12-week study of tacrolimus ointment for the treatment of atopic dermatitis in pediatric patients. *J Am Acad Dermatol* 2001; 44(Suppl):S47–57

55. Kapp A, Papp K, Bingham A, *et al.* Long-term management of atopic dermatitis in infants with topical pimecrolimus, a non-steroidal anti-inflamma-tory drug. *J Allergy Clin Immunol* 2002; 110:277–84

56. Luger T, Van Leent EJ, Graeber M, *et al.* SDZ ASM 981: an emerging safe and effective treatment for atopic dermatitis. *Br J Dermatol* 2001; 144:788–94

57. Stadler JF, Fleury M, Sourisse M, *et al.* Local steroid therapy and bacterial skin flora in atopic dermatitis. *Br J Dermatol* 1994, 131: 536–40

58. Remitz A, Kyllonen H, Granlund H, *et al.* Tacrolimus ointment reduces staphylococcal colonisation of atopic dermatitis lesions. *J Allergy Clin Immunol* 2001; 107:196–7

59. Krutmann JT, Morita A. Phototherapy for atopic dermatitis. In Bieber T, Leung DYM, eds. *Atopic Dermatitis.* New York: Marcel Dekker, 2002:501–18

60. Grundmann-Kollman M, Podda M, Ochsendorf F. Mycophenolate mofetil is effective in the treatment of atopic dermatitis. *Arch Dermatol* 2001; 137:870–3

61. Hanifin JM, Schneider LC, Leung DY, *et al.* Recombinant interferon gamma therapy for atopic dermatitis. *J Am Acad Dermatol* 1993; 28:189–97

62. Van der Briggelaar AHJ, Van Ree R, Rodriques LC, *et al.* Decreased atopy in children infected with *Schistoma haematobuim:* a role for parasite induced IL-10. *Lancet* 2000; 356:1723–7

63. Leung DYM, Sampson HA, Yunginger JW, *et al.* Effect of anti-IgE therapy in patients with peanut allergy. *N Engl J Med* 2003; 348: 986–93

Index

aciclovir 69
acrodermatitis enteropathica 76
acute eczema 19, 37
adhesins 29
adhesion molecules 21
adolescents,
    clinical features in 38
    juvenile plantar dermatosis in 59, 60
adults,
    clinical features in 38
    examples of eczema in 50–56
aeroallergens 28, 79
age,
    features related to 38
    incidence and 13, 15
    onset and 35
    remission and 15
    topical corticosteroid use and 81
air pollutants 31
allergens,
    breast-feeding 27
    food 27
    peanuts 27
    role in eczema 12
    skin response to 22
    tests 27
      for food allergies 27
allergic conjunctivitis 11
allergic rhinitis 11,12
    incidence with eczema 16, 63
    links with eczema 12
    mast cells in 23
allergy, genetics of 17
animal dander 28, 79
ankles 47
antecubital fossa 46, 50
anterior neck folds 11
anthroposophic lifestyle 32
anti-depressants 79
antibodies, monoclonal 86
antigen-presenting cells 23
antigens,
    avoidance of food antigens during pregnancy 78
    dietary 33
    in breast milk 27
    in food 27
antimicrobial peptide down-regulation in eczema 31
antiviral drugs 69
arms,

antecubital fossa involvement 46, 50
    in adult 50
    in infants 42
    lichenification on 48
asteatotic eczema 72, 73
asthma 11, 12
    incidence in eczema 16, 63
      increased 14
    links with eczema 12
    mast cells in 23
atopen 11
atopic diathesis 17
atopic keratoconjunctivitis 66
atopic syndrome 12
atopiform eczema 11
autoantigens 28
azathioprine 85

bacteria,
    antistaphylococcal treatment 84
    infections with 66
    role in eczema 28
    see also Staphylococcus;
      Streptococcus
bathing 77
blood findings in eczema 21
breast, eczema on 54
breast-feeding 33
    role in eczema 27
    role in management 78

Candida albicans 30
cathelicidins 30
central cubital fossa 48
cheilitis 11, 54
children,
    clinical features in 38
    examples of eczema in 44–49
    juvenile plantar dermatosis in 59
chromosome 1q21 18
chromosome 3p24–22 18
chromosome 3q14 18
chromosome 3q21 18, 25
chromosome 5q31 18, 25
chromosome 5q35 18
chromosome 6p 18
chromosome 6q12 26
chromosome 11q13 18, 25

chromosome 12q 18
chromosome 13q13 18
chromosome 13q14 18, 25
chromosome 14q 18
chromosome 15q14–15 18
chromosome 16q 18
chromosome 17qtel 18
chromosome 17q11 26
chromosome 17q15 18
chromosome 17q21 18
chromosome 17q25 18
chromosome 18q21 18
chromosome 20p 18
chromosome linkages to eczema 18
chronic eczema 19, 20, 37
climate 77
    cold 33
    therapy 85
clinical features 35–70
clothing 77
conjunctivitis
    allergic 11, 67
    recurrent 11
contact eczema 72, 73, 74
corticosteroids,
    intralesional 83
    systemic 85
    topical 80
      age and use of 81
      method of use 81
      side-effects of use 82
      site and use of 81
      strength of 81
creams 80
crusting 35, 36
    in infant 39, 40
      of knees 43
      severe 40
    on adult neck 53
Cushingoid features 83
cutaneous lymphocyte antigen 29, 30
cyclosporin 85
cytokines,
    antimicrobial peptides and 30
    blood findings in eczema 21
    eosinophil stimulation by 23
    production in skin 22
    use in management 86

dander 28, 79
Dead Sea Center 85
definitions,
    atopic 11
    dermatitis cf eczema 11
    extrinsic cf intrinsic 12
    variations in literature 15
Dennie-Morgan infraorbital fold 11, 63, 65
dermatitis cf eczema 11
detergents 33
diagnosis 71–76
    clinical criteria of Hanifin and Rajka 11

clinical criteria of Williams 11
diet,
    avoidance of food antigens during pregnancy 78
    dietary antigens 33
    eczema and 27
    maternal 33
    probiotic 79
    role in management 78
differential diagnosis 71–76
discoid eczema 72
discoid papular eczema 59, 62
domicile, role in eczema 13
dry skin 11, 12, 26
    causes 26
    skin function and 26

ears, eczema on 54, 58
eczema,
    bacteria and 28
    benefits to management 33
    candidate genes 25
    cf dermatitis 11
    clinical criteria 11
    clinical features 35–70
    definitions 11
    differential diagnosis 71–76
    epidemiology 13
    etiological factors 32
    etiology 25, 25
    food intolerance and 27
    genetics 17
    histology 19–21
    HLA system and 17
    infantile 12
    inflammatory cells in 23
    loci for 18
    natural history 15
    pathogenesis 19–24
    possible genetic abnormalities in 26
    T-helper-type responses in 22
    tests for 27
    triggers for 33
eczema herpeticum 69, 70
eczema vaccinatum 69
edema 35
emollients 77
emotional factors 33
enterotoxin B 30
environmental factors 13
environmental pollution 31
eosinophils 23
epidemiology 13–14
erosions 36
erythema 11
    confluent 42
    on back 41
erythrodermia 55
etiology 25
    abnormal skin barrier 26
    genetics 25
    summary of factors 32

excoriations,
    in adult 51
    in antecubital fossa 46
    in infants 39, 43
    on hands of child 44
    on legs 44, 48
exocytosis 19
eyelids,
    contact eczema on 74
    in adult 52

face,
    confluent eczema on neck and 55
    in adult 52
    in infants 39, 40
    lichenification on 52
    secondary infection of 45, 49
    Staphylococcus aureus infection of 45
famciclovir 69
family history 11
    and incidence, 17
feet, juvenile plantar dermatosis 59, 60
fibronectin 29
fissures 37
    on fingers, 61
FK 506 83
flexural involvement 12
food allergens 27
food antigen avoidance during pregnancy 78
food intolerance 11
    test for food allergies 27
fungi,
    antifungal treatment 84
    infections with 66
    role in eczema 30

genetics,
    candidate genes 25
    chromosome linkages to eczema 18
    family studies 17
    genome screens 18
    HLA system and eczema 17
    maternal effect 18
    of atopy 9
    possible abnormalities in eczema 26
    twin studies 17
genome screens 18
glucocorticosteroids 80
gluteal folds 47

hands,
    atopic eczema on 59, 60, 61
    excoriations on 44
    fissures on 61
    in infants 43
hay fever, *see under* allergic rhinitis
herpes simplex virus 11
    incidence of warts in eczema patients 69
high-affinity receptor for IgE 18
histology 19–21

hobbies 15
house dust mites 28, 33
human -defensins 30
human lymphocyte antigen (HLA) system, role in eczema 17
hygiene hypothesis 9, 32
hyperkeratosis 35
    of foot sole 37 ;
hyperkinesis 79
hyperpigmentation 55, 56
hypersensitivity type IV 21
hypertrophic lichen planus 75
hypnosis 79
hypopigmentation 56

ichthyosis vulgaris 11, 66, 68
immediate skin test (type I) reactivity 11
immune response 22
immune system
    down-regulation of antimicrobial peptides 31
    innate 30
immunoglobulin E (IgE),
    antibodies,
        blood findings in eczema 21
        chromosome linkages 18
        role in eczema 11,12
    high-affinity receptor 18
        gene for 25
    levels in diseases 24
    levels in eczema 24
    monoclonal antibody to 86
    receptors 22
    mast cells and 23
    -specific antibodies,
        Staphylococcus aureus infection and 28
        tests for 27
immunopathogenesis 21
incidence 9, 13, 31
    age and 13
    family history and 17
    increasing 13
    industrialization and 13
industrialization, 13
infantile eczema 12
infants,
    clinical features in 38
    examples of eczema in 39–44
    seborrheic eczema in 71, 72
infections, 11
    antistaphylococcal treatment 84
    antifungal treatment 84
    antiviral treatment 84
    bacterial 66
    facial 45, 49
    fungal 66
    leg 45
    viral 69
inflammatory cells 23
inheritance 17
interferon- ,
    blood findings in eczema 21
    production in eczema 22

interleukins,
    blood findings in eczema 21
    locus for interleukin-4 receptor 26
    production in eczema 22
intolerances,
    food 11
    wool 11
intralesional corticosteroids 83
itching 11, 38

juvenile plantar dermatosis 59, 60

keratoconjunctivitis 67
    atopic 66
keratoconus 66, 68
keratosis pilaris 11, 63, 64
knees,
    excoriations in adult 51
    in infants 43
    popliteal fossa involvement 45, 47

legs,
    excoriations on 48
      and crusting on 44
    in child 47
    in infants 41, 42
LEKTI 25
lichen simplex 20, 59, 62
lichenification 11, 35, 37
    facial 52
    in black child 49
    in popliteal fossa 50
    on arms 48
    pigmentation loss after 57
lifestyle 13
    anthroposophic 32
linearity, increased 63, 65
lips,
    contact eczema on 73, 74
    eczema on 54, 57
loci,
    for asthma 18
    for eczema 18,18
    for psoriasis 18
lotions 80

Malassezia furfur 30
management 77–86
    aeroallergens 79
    animal dander 79
    antifungal treatment 84
    antiviral treatment 84
    bathing 77
    biological agents 86
    breast-feeding 78
    climate 77
      climate therapy 85
    clothing 77
    corticosteroids,
      intralesional 83

    systemic 85
    topical 80
    delayed weaning 78
    diet 78
    emollients 77
    food antigen avoidance in pregnancy 78
    future developments in 86
    investigations 80
    pimecrolimus 83
    probiotics 79
    psychotherapy 79
    Staphylococcus aureus infection 84
    systemic treatment 85
    tacrolimus 83
    topical preparations 80
    ultraviolet light 84
mast cells 23
maternal effect 18
micropapular eruptions 63
migraine incidence with eczema 66
mild eczema 36
    in infant 39
molds 28
molluscum contagiosum 69
mycophenolate mofetil 86

natural history 15–16
neck,
    confluent eczema on face and 55
    in adult 53
    reticulate pigmentation on 54, 57
Netherton's syndrome 25, 75
neuropeptides 33
nitrogen oxides 32

occupation 15
ointments 80
orbital darkening 11

Paget's disease 54
pallor 11, 63
patch tests 28
pathogenesis 19–24
peanuts 27
peri-auricular eczema 54
perifollicular accentuation 11
pharmacological abnormalities 32
PHF11 25
pigmentation,
    altered 54
    hyperpigmentation 55, 56
    hypopigmentation 56
    loss after lichenification 57
    reticulate on neck 54, 57
pimecrolimus 83
pinna, eczema on 54, 58
pityriasis alba 11, 59, 62
Pityrosporum orbiculare 66
plantar dermatosis, juvenile 59, 60
plaques 37

pollens 28
pollution 9, 31, 33
popliteal fossa 45, 47
    lichenification in 50
pregnancy, avoidance of food antigens during 78
probiotics 32, 33, 79
prognosis 15
    indicators of 15
prurigo nodularis 59, 64
pruritus 11
psoriasis 75, 76
    cf histology of eczema 21
    loci for 18
psychotherapy 79
purpura and topical corticosteroid use 82

radioallergoabsorbent tests 27
RANTES 26
relapsing course 11
reticulate pigmentation on neck 54, 57
rhinitis (allergic) 11
    incidence with eczema 16, 63
    links with eczema 12
    mast cells in 23
risk of development 15

satellite lesions 48
scabies 75, 76
scaling 35, 36
    in adult 50, 53
    in infant 39, 39, 42
        on scalp and back 41
scratching,
    chronic eczema and 20
    Staphylococcus aureus infection and 29
seborrheic eczema 71, 72
sex 35
shiny foot syndrome 59, 60
side-effects,
    pimecrolimus 84
    topical corticosteroids 82
    topical tacrolimus 83
sites,
    in adolescents 38
    in adults 38
    in children 38
    in infants 38
    topical corticosteroid use and 81
skin,
    barrier function 26
    colonization by *Staphylococcus aureus* 29
    pallor 63
    see also dry skin
    thinning and topical corticosteroid use 82
skin-prick tests 27
smallpox 69
SPINKS 25
spongiosis 19
Staphylococcus aureus 11, 28
    appearance of infections 66

facial infection 45
infection in infants 38
management of infections 66
role in eczema 30
superantigens and 29
T-cell activation by 29
treatment of 84
Streptococci 28
stress 33
striae and topical corticosteroid use 82
subacute eczema 19, 36
subcapsular cataracts 11
sulfur dioxide 32
superantigens,
    effects of 30
    pathogenesis and 29
symmetry 54
systemic treatment,
    azathioprine 85
    corticosteroids 85
    cyclosporin 85
    mycophenolate mofetil 86

T-cells 23
    activation by *Staphylococcus aureus* 29
    clones 27
T-helper type cells 21
T-helper-type responses,
    fungi and 30
    hygiene hypothesis 32
    in eczema 22
    Staphylococcus aureus and 29
tacrolimus 83
telangiectasia and topical corticosteroid use 83
tests 80
    IgE-specific antibodies 27
    patch 28
    radioallergoabsorbent 27
    skin-prick 27
thighs 47
Toll-like receptors 30
topical corticosteroids 80–83
topical preparations 80
treatment, *see under* management
Trichophyton rubrum 66
trunk, in infants 40, 41
twin studies in eczema 17
type IV hypersensitivity 21

ultraviolet light 84
urbanization 9
urticaria, incidence with eczema 66

vaccination 32
vaccinia virus 69
vascular abnormalities 32
vascular cell adhesion molecule 21
virus,
    antiviral treatment 84
    eczema herpeticum 70

infections with 69

warts 60, 69
weaning 33
    delayed 78
weather 77
    climate therapy 85
    cold 33
weeping 37
white dermographism 63, 65
Wiskott-Aldrich syndrome 75
wool intolerance 11
wrists, symmetrical involvement 46

xeroderma 63
xerosis, *see under* dry skin

T - #0345 - 101024 - C0 - 280/208/6 [8] - CB - 9781842142363 - Gloss Lamination